FAMILIES AND LARGER SYSTEMS

THE GUILFORD FAMILY THERAPY SERIES
ALAN S. GURMAN, EDITOR

FAMILIES AND LARGER SYSTEMS
A Family Therapist's Guide through the Labyrinth

EVAN IMBER-BLACK

THE GUILFORD PRESS
New York   London

To Lascelles W. Black
my husband, my partner, my model
of compassionate and effective
work in larger systems

© 1988 The Guilford Press
A Division of Guilford Publications, Inc.
72 Spring Street, New York, NY 10012

Printed in the United States of America

Last digit is print number: 9 8 7 6 5 4 3

Library of Congress Cataloging-in-Publication Data

Imber-Black, Evan.
　Families and larger systems.

　(The Guilford family therapy series)
　Includes bibliographies and index.
　1. Family psychotherapy. 2. Family. 3. Social
institutions. I. Title. II. Series. [DNLM: 1. Family.
2. Family Therapy. 3. Social Environment.
WM 430.5.F2 I32f]
RC488.5.I43　1988　　　616.89'156　　　87-31343
ISBN 0-89862-100-3　　ISBN 0-89862-109-7 (pbk.)

Acknowledgments

My own fascination with families and larger systems reaches back to growing up in a family where the larger systems of synagogue and Jewish service organizations blended into the daily lives of my father, Elmer Imber, and my mother, Dena Imber, shaping our family's organization and relationships to the outside world. As a child, I was imbued with a commitment to purposive action in larger systems whose raison d'etre was the expansion of justice and compassion.

When I was twenty, I began teaching in an inner-city high school in Chicago. My own oddysey into public-sector larger systems began in my weekly summons to the assistant principal's office. He would scream at me for what, in retrospect, was my Don Quixote-like behavior in a larger system that was filled with racism and classism, and I, in turn, would cry, leave his office, break another "rule," and be summoned again. I can only thank him now for what proved to be an introduction to the interactional regularities in larger systems, and for unwittingly encouraging my search for more effective responses.

My academic interest in families and larger systems was nurtured in my doctoral work at the University of Pittsburgh, under the competent mentorship of Dr. Canice Connors, who taught me to combine scholarly interests with action in consultation to larger systems.

The present work took shape in three distinct professional and geographic settings. What has ultimately become the family–larger system assessment model began in my work as director of the Family Therapy specialty area at the University of Massachusetts, Amherst. From 1977 to 1982, I was blessed with doctoral students in the family–larger system seminar who were committed to developing excellent public sector models of practice, many of whom became my colleagues. Dr. Lee Bell's work examining change in public schools, Dr. Linda Webb-Watson's work examining families and welfare systems, Dr. Jill Harkaway's work looking at the interaction of families, overweight, and the larger systems organized to address weight problems, Dr. Dusty Miller's work examining alcoholic families and larger systems, and Dr. Frank Harrell's work looking at family–larger system triads all contributed to the development of my own thinking and practice. Dr. Stephen Bloomfield and Sergio Pirrota demonstrated the efficacy of the concepts in the administration of large public sector systems. Dr. Margaret Kierstein and Dr. Serena Lurie helped test many of the early ideas in a specialized foster care project in rural Western Massachusetts. All of the above-named people affirmed the validity of a family–larger system perspective.

The Franklin County Mental Health Center, the Berkshire Mental Health Center, the Pittsfield, Massachusetts public school family therapy project, and the University of Massachusetts LIFT project were all instrumental in providing practice centers for the genesis of the present work. While the many participants are too numerous to mention, I trust that they know that they have my appreciation for their support and their willingness to explore the family–larger system terrain with me.

Further developments in family–larger system interviewing and intervention design were made at the Family Therapy Program in the Department of Psychiatry, University of Calgary, Alberta, Canada. I especially want to thank Dr. Karl Tomm for designing an atmosphere that encouraged clinical creativity and curiosity, and for his ongoing support of my family–larger system inquiry, including my clinical work and my writing. I also want to thank the clinical and academic staff, especially Dr. Gary Sanders, Ms. Maria Bakaitis, Ms. Karine Rietgens, Dr. Alan Parry, Ms. Joanne Hall, Dr. M. J. Ferrier, Dr. Dusty Miller, and Mr. Bill Stewart for their participation in the development of this work in the family–larger system seminar, and in our collaboration on difficult family–larger system cases, which enabled further refinement of this work. My deep appreciation is expressed to Ms. Myrna Fraser, Administrative Assistant at the Family Therapy Program, for her loyalty, her friendship, and her abiding interest in my work. I thank the late Dr. Sebastian Littman, who, as chairman of the department of psychiatry, made himself available for ongoing discussions of this work, and Dr. Michael Entwisle who supported the application of the concepts both at the province-wide Alberta Mental Health Services, and in the training of psychiatric residents as mental health consultants. I also thank Dr. Lorraine Wright for her colleagueship and her encouragement of the work during my time in Calgary.

The connections between family–larger system interaction and the wider social context and the opportunity to try the ideas in a poor and urban primary health care setting were made possible by my affiliation with the Residency Program in Social Medicine, Montefiore Medical Center, Bronx, New York, under the leadership of Dr. Robert Massad.

Here I have met colleagues and residents whose commitment to public sector practice has affirmed my own belief in a family–larger system perspective. In particular, I thank Ms. Eliana Korin and Dr. Celestine Fulchon for struggling with me to translate the ideas in ways that are relevant to primary care residents.

The material on women, families, and larger systems began to take shape at the first Stonehenge Conference. I thank Ms. Monica McGoldrick, Dr. Froma Walsh, and Dr. Carol Anderson for providing me with this opportunity, and all of the women who participated and encouraged this aspect of my work. I especially thank Ms. Betty Carter for welcoming this element of my work via my affiliation with the Family Institute of Westchester, and for her abiding friendship.

The material on ritual interventions with families and larger systems rises out of my decade-long collaboration with Dr. Janine Roberts and Dr. Dick Whiting. I especially thank them for their steady faith in my work and for their caring friendship.

I had many nurturing discussions of this work with Mr. Pat Lenon, the Canadian Western regional director of the L'Arche Community. He helped me refine my thinking regarding the applicability of these ideas to persons with handicaps, their families, larger systems, and the wider social context.

I want to thank those people who looked at earlier drafts of the manuscript, including Dr. Don Brown, Dr. Rich Simon, and especially Dr. Joel Feiner for our ongoing discussions of the applicability of the concepts to complex public-sector practice and training. I thank Dr. Alan Gurman very much for encouraging me to write the book, and for his editorial assistance. I also want to thank Dr. Don Efron for enabling me to establish a receptivity to many of the ideas in this book as guest editor of a special issue of the *Journal of Strategic and Systemic Therapies*.

I have been extremely fortunate to be able to develop all of the ideas set forth in this work through my direct involvement with families and helpers in diverse settings in the United States, Canada, and Western Europe. The generosity of families and helpers in allowing me to enter their lives as a therapist or consultant led to the clinical material available in this book. Their names have, of course, been changed for reasons of confidentiality. I thank them deeply, and wish them to know that the concepts were co-created by my involvement with them.

I thank Ms. Shelly Hall who typed the first draft of the first five chapters. I express my deep appreciation to Ms. Madeline Bunce, who typed and re-typed the entire manuscript. Both of these women endured my idiosyncratic methods of making revisions, never complained, and kept me smiling.

Finally, I want to give my appreciation to my loving family. They have been patient regarding the loss of our leisure time together, and have supported my work in every way I can imagine. My son, Jason, assisted me instrumentally by facilitating my relationship to the word processor, convinced me that cursing at it would make it user unfriendly, and supported me with his love and concern. My daughter, Jennifer, who faces her own developmental disabilities with courage, has been and remains my most personal reason for the present work. Her resolve and her caring as she navigates complex larger systems sustains me. My stepdaughter, Naomi, entered my life as this book began, and has added to the richness of my existence by her endless curiosity about the world around her. My husband, Lascelles Black, continually demonstrates the caring and respectful work that is possible in larger systems. Our ongoing discussions of our mutual work during the writing of this book, and his loving support of my work always made me know that what I was doing mattered to him. I thank him for this special gift.

Evan Imber-Black

Foreword

Family therapists hardly ever encounter a family whose experience is not profoundly influenced by larger system involvement, whether it be the health care system, the school system, the legal system, or a social agency. And yet most family therapists operate as if families existed in a vacuum. Family therapy grew up in reaction to the myopia of the psychoanalytic movement, which tended to neglect or ignore the profundity of their patients' basic context: the family. But family therapists have had great difficulty moving beyond the level of the family to larger systemic levels. Now Dr. Evan Imber-Black has provided us with a brilliant guide for using our "systemic" understanding to consider families in their larger contexts.

Dr. Imber-Black is unique in the field of family therapy in directing our attention to the larger social systems in which families are embedded and in providing us with useful guidelines for conceptualizing and responding to the patterns that develop between families and public agencies. While others, particularly in the field of social work, have long paid attention to welfare, health, and other human services in meeting the needs of families, Imber-Black provides us with a metaperspective, clearly defining the typical problems that develop between systems, as well as the ways that "helping" systems often contribute to the very problems they were established to resolve.

Dr. Imber-Black discusses a central myth that pervades the sociocultural context in North America that holds that the nuclear family is an independent sanctuary, in need of no outside help or support. As she says, this myth forms a potent backdrop for all that occurs between families and larger systems, since families do indeed need all sorts of outside support. Yet they often are made to feel inadequate and "sick" for having such needs. Dr. Imber-Black discusses with outstandingly clear and recognizable examples the vicious cycles that often develop between families and larger systems vis-à-vis each other that limit creative, effective solutions. She describes the binds that agencies often put families in by which they are seen as "sick" if they admit to having problems and "sick" if they do not, or expect families to act open to treatment, when they are, in fact, being coerced into it and when their very openness may subject them to being penalized by the agency.

Dr. Imber-Black also examines the crucial issues of labeling, stigma, and secrets regarding families' relationships with larger systems. She defines situations in which a consultant can intervene to relabel a family member, detoxify a stigmatizing condition, or work to shift the boundaries marked by secrets that have become problematic for a family or between a family and outsiders.

One of the most important topics touched upon by Dr. Imber-Black regarding this important subject is the interface of gender with larger system issues, since, as she says, "Larger systems are the transmitters of our culture's assumptions and fundamental values regarding human beings, their need for care, focus of blame, and responsibility for change. If they remain unexamined or unquestioned, it is easy for larger systems to support a patriarchal process reflective of the culture at large." Dr. Imber-Black offers some excellent examples of these problems, including the important subject of consulting on gender issues within the larger system, which itself reproduces the gender hierarchies of the wider culture. In spite of her clarity, she provides no cookbook answers that will make the problems she describes vanish. There are no simple answers for these problems. She is to be applauded for addressing these issues head on, without suggesting that we can make them disappear through a consultation.

Families and Larger Systems should be required reading for all family therapy trainees and all those working in public agencies—at whatever level. Because it questions the assumptions of our organizational practice, it provides a crucial framework within which we can begin to consider family therapy practice as more than a fad. Throughout her book Dr. Imber-Black raises questions for agency personnel to consider: Who is defining the problem as a problem? How does each participant in the situation define the problem? What is the overall agenda of each system? How is the agency viewed by the family? How is it viewed by the public? We need to develop this broader perspective as a framework for all our work with families. Dr. Imber-Black has gone a very long way in lighting our path.

Monica McGoldrick

Contents

CHAPTER 1

Families and Larger Systems: An Often Troubled Terrain

Family therapy originated with the idea that an individual's problems begin to make a different kind of sense when examined in the context of the nuclear and extended family. That idea can be expanded into an even more complex meaningful system, composed of individuals, family, and larger systems, existing in a wider social context that shapes and guides mutual expectations, specific interactions, and outcomes. The skills required in systemic assessment of and intervention with families make the family therapist particularly suited for work at the macrosystemic level.

The often problematic interaction of families and larger systems requires attention from the therapist seeking to intervene with families while maintaining viable relationships in the broad professional community. The following vignette gives a sample of the complexity of the family–larger system interaction.

BRIEF EXAMPLE: WHEN MORE IS LESS

The following group assembled to determine the immediate future of a 13-year-old girl, Marla: one child psychiatrist, one consulting psychiatrist, a psychologist engaged in marital therapy with the girl's parents, a child-welfare worker, a child-care worker from the detention center, two recent foster parents from whose home the girl had run, a resource teacher, a school psychologist, two residential treatment managers, two directors of a residential treatment cottage, a family therapist from residential treatment, and a Big Sister. Marla and her parents were also at the meeting. During the introductions, when Marla's turn came, she looked around at the assembly, smiled, and said, "And I'm Marla, and I'm the star of this show!"

A variety of themes and issues emerged during the course of this meeting, which involved five times as many professionals as there were members of the family. The present nuclear family had been involved with professional helping systems for over a quarter of a century and in three different states. Conflictual interaction with professional helpers occurred also in the parents' families of origin.

Presenting problems included parental alcoholism, neglect charges, marital conflict, and symptomatic behavior in each of three children, including school problems, delinquency, and drug abuse.

The range of outsiders* included psychiatrists, pediatricians, welfare workers, probation officers, school personnel, foster parents, marital and family therapists, psychologists, residential treatment staff, and paraprofessional community workers. This meeting was the first occasion where all of the helpers had met one another. An oscillating pattern of great optimism about progress and change, followed by deep pessimism and despair, marked both family and helpers. Such optimism emerged when any new helper entered the family sphere and was maintained for a brief period until family and helper became frustrated with one another, when a new helper would be enlisted. At the meeting, the family expressed a strong sense of "good" helpers and "bad" helpers. The helpers, in turn, were sharply divided regarding their views of the family, with some seeing a "good" family and others seeing a "bad" one. A consensus between family and helpers emerged only on the topic of Marla's future. All agreed that she would continue to have serious problems and that involvement with professionals would continue to be necessary. The family and helpers formed a macrosystem marked by predictable patterns, familiar processes, a shared "identified patient," and pessimism regarding viable change. Both family and helpers, however, were caught up in this macrosystem in ways that prevented all concerned from appreciating the patterns in ways that would make change possible. The connection between family and larger systems had a life of its own, one that continued across generations while individual helpers were replaced by other helpers.

Families and larger systems frequently become engaged with one another in unfortunate ways, ways that impede growth and development in family members and contribute to cynicism and burnout among helpers. All too frequently, little attention is paid to the patterns that emerge between families and larger systems, resulting in the replication and reification of unsatisfactory relationships at multiple levels.

*The term *outsiders* will be used interchangeably with *larger systems representatives* and *helpers*.

FAMILIES TALK ABOUT HELPERS: A FEW
BRIEF EXAMPLES

1. In an interview of a single-parent family with an adolescent son who refused to go to school, the following interchange occurred:

CONSULTANT: (*to son*) Suppose we stopped all these efforts of therapy, counseling, truant officer, medication, et cetera, how do you think your mother would do?

SON: (*crying*) She wouldn't be hurting so much.

CONSULTANT: Are you saying all these outside efforts make it worse for her?

SON: Yes. She figures if she has to get help, it means she's helpless, and she feels worse.

A short while later, the son also indicated that stopping all helping efforts would be hardest on his mother, thus illustrating a major difficulty in the family–larger system relationship, whereby the mother feels more and more helpless in the face of more and more help yet is unable to extricate herself due to this very sense of helplessness. Second on the son's list of people who would have the hardest time if outside help were to stop was the school counselor, the primary facilitator of the entry of new helpers.

2. During a consultation to a mother who was being given advice to hospitalize her child by a school psychologist, while simultaneously being given advice not to hospitalize her child by a family therapist, the following interchange occurred:

CONSULTANT: You're in a tough spot right now.

MOTHER: As usual. I'm in the middle.

CONSULTANT: What do you mean?

MOTHER: Well—whoever is at one moment helping us is on one side, and my child is always on the other side, and me, I'm in the middle, caught between the two. Now it's even worse, because I'm also in the middle between the counselor and the therapist!

3. During an interview of a family warmly engaged with several helpers, with no hint of change, the following interchange occurred:

CONSULTANT: Who has helped you the most?

FATHER: Oh, it's a combination of all of them. They've been terrific!

CONSULTANT: Who's been the most helpful?

DAUGHTER: [sister of the identified patient] (*starts to identify the proba-tion officer and then corrects herself*) I mean, really, it's a combination of all of them.

CONSULTANT: Has any of the help you've received been effective in solv-ing the problems between you and your daughter?

FATHER: Well no, but they all have such good ideas!

CONSULTANT: [later in the interview] You said you think your daughter will be fine and quite successful in 5 years. Will she do that on her own or with professional help?

FATHER: Oh, on her own! She's very stubborn. The more help you give her, the more determined she is to prove she doesn't need it!

All of the other family members agreed with the father regarding the efficacy of help for the identified patient and then rushed to reassure the helpers that they were loved and appreciated for all of their efforts.

4. During an interview focusing on previous help, the following emerged:

MOTHER: I took the children to see Dr. M. during my divorce, because Alan was acting up so much. Then, all of the sessions were spent modi-fying *my* behavior. I felt very put down. Later, we went to the Crisis Center because Stu ran away [This running away was directly linked to Stu being molested by a Big Brother.], and they gave me a sheet on "mothering skills" and insisted Stu was running away because I was remarrying!

5. During an exploration of intergenerational attitudes towards help in a family engaged with medical, legal, and therapeutic profession-als for 7 years, the following information was shared:

MOTHER: My family is Ukrainian. It's a little hard for them to understand all that's happening to us.

CONSULTANT: When there was a problem in your family how would people solve it? Who would they turn to?

MOTHER: Oh, we'd never tell outsiders! That was a rule—you solved things yourself!

CONSULTANT: How do they feel now about your involvement with out-side professionals?

MOTHER: Oh, they don't know! We'd never tell them—they would think it's just awful!

CONSULTANT: If they did know, what might they say about how things have gone?

MOTHER: Well, I guess they wouldn't be too surprised that none of it's worked.

6. During an interview with a single-parent family who self-referred because of problems remaining after a 5-year history of sexual abuse of a teenage girl by her stepfather, an inquiry was made into prior help the family had received.

MOTHER: After she told me that this had been going on, I went with her to a counselor in our town. This was before I left him.

CONSULTANT: What was that experience like?

DAUGHTER: It wasn't too helpful. He just said that my stepfather was having a "quirk" and that I should put a lock on my door. He didn't think I needed counseling. I don't think he really believed me.

HELPERS TALK ABOUT FAMILIES AND OTHER HELPERS: A FEW BRIEF EXAMPLES

1. In interviewing several family therapists regarding their most difficult cases, a variation of the following was heard again and again:

THERAPIST: The cases that make me want to head for the hills are the ones where the family is seeing lots of professionals. I just don't know what to do, and it never turns out well. Usually I'll try to coordinate our efforts, but it almost never works, and I often end up angry with the other professionals and feel quite incompetent.

2. A probation officer, whose mandate is to find appropriate services for her clients, stated, "Often I'll recommend various types of counseling or therapy for my clients and their families. But it seems the families feel blamed when I do this, and the therapists treat me like I'm part of the problem!"

3. A family therapist and a school counselor were involved with the same family, regarding a boy who refused to go to school. Their views towards each other and the constraints of their contexts became apparent in the following:

SCHOOL COUNSELOR: My superior thinks Jim has a serious psychiatric problem and needs to be hospitalized. But the family sessions are only held once every 2 or 3 weeks—the seriousness of the matter just isn't being recognized. I stop in to see the family almost daily now.

FAMILY THERAPIST: I don't think Jim has a psychiatric problem. The school counselor is overreacting! Jim's a stubborn young man with some very important reasons for choosing not to grow up right now. I've been working towards normalizing this situation.

4. A child-welfare worker, who had spent a lot of time hearing the side of a 14-year-old boy in his dispute with his foreign-born parents and whose efforts were seen by the family as an insulting intrusion, said, "This family is just going to have to learn that their son is Canadian, not Greek! They can't keep doing things the way they would do them in Greece. I think their son is right to not want to live with them anymore!"

5. A family therapist sought a consultation for a case that involved him, a welfare worker, a probation officer, and a residential treatment program. Progress in the case was stalled. The family expressed a great liking for the family therapist and the welfare worker, while expressing great displeasure with the probation officer and the residential program. In discussing the case the family therapist said, "I like this family very much—maybe too much. I actually feel like a member of the family, and I know I don't want them to regard me the way they regard some of the other helpers. I have a feeling I'm going to be working with them forever!"

The foregoing vignettes are only a few examples of the range and depth of problems that can arise between families and larger systems as they interact with one another. When families and helpers are invited to talk about their experiences with each other, such problems often emerge, usually within a framework of blame. Families may experience themselves as coerced, patronized, trapped, or otherwise served poorly by professionals, despite good intentions. At the same time, professionals may experience themselves as misunderstood, unappreciated, and criticized by particular families and other professionals. Often what is missing is a cogent analysis of the *meaningful system* that is formed when families and larger systems come together and create patterns that either facilitate or impede problem resolution and human development.

This book addresses the issue of families and larger systems from a number of vantage points, including the ways that families and larger systems become engaged with and disengaged from one another, historical and cultural imperatives affecting this mutual engagement, larger system mandates and constraints, expectations on both sides, and emergent patterns and themes. The material in this book is the culmination of a decade of work with families and larger systems. All of the case examples are from my clinical, consulting, and research interviews with families who have been intensely involved with larger systems, and with helpers from larger systems who have worked with such families. An assessment model for understanding the complex phenomenon of families and larger systems and a variety of interviewing formats and intervention possibilities are included and illustrated by clinical case material. While this work focuses on families and larger systems, many of the principles pertain as well to individual clients or couples who engage with professional helpers. The larger systems addressed in this work are primarily public-sector helping and human service systems, including hospitals, schools, clinics, welfare, probation, residential treatment, geriatric services, and so on; however, the issues discussed can also apply to other larger systems that effect families, such as religious institutions or work.

CONTEXT OF THE PRESENT WORK

The problems of families and larger systems have been highlighted in a small but growing literature that has concerned itself primarily with problems arising between families and specific kinds of larger systems such as hospitals, schools, probation, or welfare, or with specific presenting problems in families and the particular treatment systems designed to address these problems. The current work seeks to go the next step by offering an heuristic model for assessing and intervening in the family–larger system relationship in ways that cut across specific larger systems and specific presenting problems.

Twenty years ago, in the family therapy field, E. H. Auerswald (1968) called attention to family–larger system interaction. In what he referred to as an "ecological systems approach," he focused on the interaction of patients, their families, and the agencies providing services.

Problematic interaction between families and hospitals was discussed by Bell and Zucker (1968–1969), who pointed to patterns of mutual avoidance and escalating distance between family members and hospital personnel who shared a common member, the patient. More recently, Harbin (1985) discussed the conflicts between families and psychiatric hospitals, describing families as primary, informal systems and hospitals as large, formal systems, who easily misunderstand each other without either system being essentially dysfunctional. Harbin's work points to the possibilities of work focusing on the strengths of each of the subsystems (e.g., hospital and family as subsystems of the larger macrosystem formed by the two) and does not deal with macrosystemic assessment and intervention.

Homeostatic patterns between families and physicians and the effect of these on family therapy outcome was pointed to by Selvini Palazzoli,

Boscolo, Cecchin, and Prata (1980b). The Milan group discussed what they called "the problem of the referring person," punctuating the issue as one caused by an "overinvolved" professional who had become "like a family member." They offered examples of strategies to address this circumstance but stopped short of conceptualizing the issue as one between family systems and larger systems.

Difficulties between families and public schools have been addressed by Aponte (1976), Imber Coppersmith (1982a, 1982b), and Coleman (1983). All three authors offer clinical descriptions of the family–school macrosystem and offer working methods that specifically address the triad formed by the family, the school, and the child.

Several authors have focused on triads and boundaries as essential concepts with which to examine families and larger systems. In "The Myth of the Multi-Problem Family," Selig (1976) reframes the issue of multiproblem families as that of families with multiple agencies involved in their lives. Harrell (1980) expands the multiagency phenomenon to a discussion of problematic triads between families and outside systems that interdicted the therapeutic progress. Harrell's research, comparing families who were involved for generations with larger systems with families who entered and exited larger systems with their problems solved, pointed to the existence of conflictual and enduring triads, between families and the larger systems, that made progress and problem resolution impossible. Schwartzman and Restivo (1985) discussed the juvenile probation system and families and highlighted ways in which the juvenile justice system mirrors the family systems of delinquent youth, particularly in triadic patterns, paradoxical messages, and lack of constraints for the juvenile. Bokos and Schwartzman (1985) examined methadone programs and indicated the many ways in which institutions, designed to solve specific problems, frequently end up perpetuating these very problems by replicating family patterns. Both of these works point to the need to carefully analyze larger treatment systems in order to avoid the replication of family patterns, but stop short of providing detailed interventions or outcomes. Similarly, Schwartzman and Kneifel (1985), in their look at a child-care system and families, discussed the problems that emerge when patterns in the larger system replicate family patterns and utilized the concepts "too richly cross-joined" and "too poorly cross-joined" as their primary organizing concepts for examining the subsystems of family and larger system and problematic interaction between the two. All three of the foregoing works added to a systemic view of families and larger systems but did not highlight assessment and intervention aimed at the macrosystemic level, nor did they provide details for the clinician seeking to decide the appropriate level of intervention (e.g., individual, dyadic, family, larger system, or macrosystemic level).

Specific presenting problems that often lead to difficulties, disappointments, and despair between families and larger systems have been discussed by a number of authors. These have studied families with handicapped members at various developmental stages (Berger, 1984; Bloomfield, Neilson, & Kaplan, 1984; Combrinck-Graham & Higley, 1984; MacKinnon & Marlett, 1984; Roberts, 1984), families with alcohol problems (Miller, 1983), and families with obesity problems (Harkaway, 1983). All point to the ways in which larger systems, designed to alleviate specific problems, in fact end up perpetuating these problems because of a lack of focus on family–larger system patterns. MacKinnon and Marlett (1984) enlarged the focus further through an examination of the historical and social context within which families with handicapped members and larger systems are embedded, including the prejudice and discrimination in this context. This sociohistorical perspective is elaborated by Imber-Black (1986d) in a brief examination of the ways in which larger systems often perpetuate sexism in their work with women clients, whose problems frequently originate from sexist social structures.

Most of the existing literature is descriptive, providing definitions of the problems that exist between families and larger systems. Some presents case material suggestive of directions for future work (Coleman, 1983; Goolishian & Anderson, 1981; Harkaway, 1983; Hoffman & Long, 1969; Imber-Black, 1986d; Imber Coppersmith, 1982a, 1983b, 1985a; Miller, 1983; Schwartzman & Kneifel, 1985; Selvini Palazzoli et al., 1980b; Tomm, Lannaman & McNamee, 1983; Webb-Woodard, & Woodard, 1983), which the present volume addresses.

The current work builds on these prior works in order to provide clinicians with pragmatic direction for assessing, interviewing, and intervening in families and larger systems in ways that may solve problems and enhance well-being for family members *and* for the professionals involved.

The seemingly intractable problems between a family and larger systems may be following a pattern that, never recognized, rigidly prescribes roles for everyone involved. For generations a family may present similar problems and grapple with similar nonsolutions.

CASE EXAMPLE: FAMILY–LARGER SYSTEM HISTORY REPEATS ITSELF

The Franklin family, consisting of two parents and two children, had a multigenerational history with larger systems. Both parents had spent major portions of their adolescence in foster care facilities, and both came from families who had little use for helpers, seeing them as "meddling, nosy, and unhelpful." The father had a history of problems with alcohol and occasionally would seek help, but with little belief in the efficacy of outside help. The mother sought individual therapy from time to time but would drop out when she sensed the therapist believed she should leave her husband. In their written reports, helpers judged the parents as "resistant, uncooperative." Thus, prior to their present engagement, the family and outside systems had established a long-standing pattern of involvement marked by mutual disappointment and disapproval (see Figure 1-1).

The parents began to have trouble with their daughter as she entered adolescence, the same developmental period when they had to leave their own families and engage with larger systems. Corey, 13, began to shoplift and abuse alcohol. In a move that was familiar to the parents from their past, they called in Child Welfare, stating they could not handle their daughter and requesting that she be placed in a foster home. Although the Child Welfare worker determined the parents' history of foster care as adolescents, this was assessed *only* as information about the family, rather than as crucial information regarding the family and larger systems in an ongoing relationship marked by repetitive patterns and fixed beliefs.

It was determined, with the parents' agreement, that they could not handle Corey, and she was placed in a residential treatment program for adolescents. She was given an individual therapist, and the family was told they must come to family therapy. Early on, the family indicated their intense displeasure at having family sessions and clearly communicated their general disdain for helping professionals. In turn, the family was seen as being uncooperative. The stage was set for troubled interaction between the family and larger systems.

About a month after Corey's arrival in residence, she returned from a weekend home visit very upset. She had fought with her parents and was very angry, especially with her father. At this juncture, the cottage staff, who were accustomed to seeing abused children, questioned Corey in this regard. She told them she was not presently abused, but that her father had molested her on two occasions when she was 11. At this juncture a number of actions ensued: (1) The residential facility notified the police and requested an investigation. (2) The parents were told that Corey could not visit home but could only have supervised visits on campus. The parents were not told the reason for the change. (3) Corey refused to talk to her individual therapist. The therapist assumed this meant Corey was keeping secrets and felt compelled to press her further, resulting in further silence and eventual sullenness on Corey's part. (4) The police did not go to the family to investigate for 2 months. During this time, conflict escalated between the family and the residence, with Corey caught in the middle. As the family became angrier, the residence made more rules limiting contact, such as listening in on Corey's telephone conversations with her parents because the parents were criticizing the residence, and shortening supervised visits. (5) The

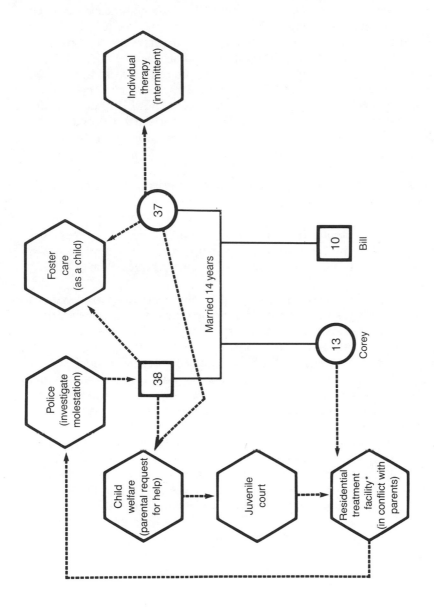

*director, cottage staff, family therapist, psychologist

Figure 1-1. The Franklin family and outside systems interaction.

11

police investigated and determined that the abuse had indeed occurred 2 years ago and had stopped. No charges were pressed. (6) The family insisted they would not discuss the matter further, while the residence insisted that sexual abuse be the topic of family therapy and, until this occurred, normal visiting could not resume. In response to this impasse, Corey's behavior deteriorated. The family blamed the residence and its rules for Corey's situation, while the residence blamed the family. Child Welfare sided with the residence, while the police sided with the family. Mutual mistrust and conflict permeated the macrosystem. (The resolution of this case is discussed in Chapter 5.)

This example raises many questions applicable to family–larger systems relationships in general.

1. What methods for understanding problematic engagement between families and larger systems enable one to see pattern, process, contextual constraints, and cocreated themes, rather than atomized blame?

2. How can a family's history of involvement with larger systems inform current practice such that repetition is avoided and new information regarding relationship options is made available?

3. How does the mandate of a particular larger system interact with family process for either a good or a troubled outcome?

4. What are common interactional regularities between families and larger systems? How can one intervene effectively in this complex process?

5. What are the effects of labeling on the family–larger system relationship?

6. What are the effects of actual secrets and presumed secrets in the family–larger system relationship?

7. What are the effects when families and multiple helpers interact? What patterns emerge? What happens to the focus of responsible action?

8. What are the effects of blurred boundaries among various components of a larger system? In particular, how can effective therapy, individual or family, be offered within larger systems whose primary mandate is social control? In what ways do larger systems reflect social, political, and economic policy toward families and towards class, ethnic, gender, and racial distinctions?

9. What are the necessary elements to create beneficial relationships between families and larger systems?

10. What are the components in training professionals to work with families and larger systems?

To grapple with these questions, this book will proceed in the format described in the following paragraphs.

Chapter 2 examines the ways in which families and larger systems become engaged with one another, including the meanings of such engagement for all concerned, the processes of initiating contact, and the often unspoken expectations for both family and helpers. The interaction between helpers' mandates and multigenerational and cultural attitudes towards particular outside systems is examined. The effects of larger-system organization and change as this reflects wider public policy and social context are discussed, particularly in reference to the multiple-helper phenomena. Referral, patterns of exit, and the "no-exit" family–larger system relationship are examined.

Chapter 3 presents an assessment model for understanding the family–larger system relationship and applies the model to a case.

Chapter 4 presents interviewing modalities for assessing and intervening in the family–larger system relationship and includes methods for inviting helpers, the role of the consultant, different formats for interviewing the family without helpers, interviewing helpers without the family, and conducting family–helper sessions.

Chapter 5 focuses on intervention design, implementation, and evaluation in the family–larger system relationship, including an examination of the context of interventions, tasks, rituals, and opinions and of the creative uses of memos and reports as interventions.

Chapter 6 describes ways to create a new, unanticipated, and effective relationship between a family and larger systems. The focus is on ongoing work with families and larger systems. Issues of labeling, stigma, and secrecy in the macrosystem are discussed. Therapist positions and the need for coaching and advocacy are exemplified.

Chapter 7 deals with women, families, and larger systems and specifically discusses women's issues as these are affected by policies and procedures of larger systems.

Chapter 8 focuses on consulting to larger systems.

CHAPTER 2

Entries, Exits, and No-Exits

All families engage with larger systems. It is mythical to posit families as self-sufficient entities, although this is a prevalent myth in Western culture today. Rather, most families are able to function in an interdependent manner with a variety of larger systems, utilizing information from these systems as material for their own growth and development. For most families such engagement proceeds in ways that are largely nonproblematic. Families send their children to school, and while they may occasionally encounter a problem with a particular teacher or another child or brief behavioral or learning problems, the relationship between most families and schools proceeds fairly smoothly. At various points in their life cycle families engage with medical personnel, both for routine health care and for specific illnesses, and while they may find a particular physician or nurse not to their liking or not meeting their needs, most often the relationships between families and health care providers do not generate unsolvable problems. Families engage with religious and cultural institutions, work settings, and other social systems, and while such outside systems may at times generate stress for families (and vice versa), most families do not become bogged down by problems with outside systems such that impasses are reached and individual and family development and well-being are *seriously* effected.

For a significant portion of the population, however, engagement with larger systems becomes problematic and remains problematic for long periods of time, taking a toll on normative development, potential, and problem solving while supporting symptomatic behavior and a narrowed sense of choice and creative capacity.

Such troubled engagement is determined by multiple causes. Studying the context of initiation of family–larger system involvement often yields explanations, as well as potential areas for subsequent intervention. Particular patterns and themes mark the entry process of relationships between families and larger systems. These include patterns and themes that lie within the family and become apparent upon engagement with larger systems, patterns and themes that lie within larger systems and become apparent upon engagement with particular families, and situations where family and larger systems make an idiosyncratic bad fit.

FAMILY PATTERNS AND THEMES AFFECTING ENTRY

Many families have a history of involvement with outsiders over several generations (Harrell, 1980; Miller, 1983). Interacting with outside professionals is a familiar way to conduct family life. Engagement with any new helper exists in a historical context of such involvement and carries with it successes and failures of such engagement, spanning decades. For some families, such engagement has been "friendly and warm" but has resulted in no fundamental change. One helper fills the place of another in a serial pattern. Such engagement may be member specific across the generations: Perhaps only the mothers become involved with outsiders, turning in one generation to a priest, in the next to a physician, and in the third to a therapist and structuring similar relationships with each—for example, succorance and support for dealing with an "aberrant" husband, who is relieved that his wife's complaints are being "handled" and that pressures on him and on the marital pair are reduced.

Or a family may be familiar with conflictual engagement with outsiders, occurring for several generations at particular developmental stages. For some families, troubled engagement ensues when children start school. For others, difficulties with outside systems ensue at the "leaving home" stage of child and family development. Outsiders may come to function in repetititve ways, either to facilitate or impede this stage of development, such that the family's familiar legacy becomes "children cannot leave home without the entry of outside systems" or, conversely, "children do *not* leave home when outside systems enter."

Still other families have multigenerational patterns of intense conflict or disappointment with larger systems, such that the entry of any new helper exists in a context of years and years of anger, blame, and mistrust between the family and outsider. The parents may feel coerced to have helpers, just as their parents felt coerced, or may simply turn to helpers because parents and grandparents did, even though help was never helpful and no one expects it to be in the present.

BRIEF EXAMPLE: A "TRIADIC" MARRIAGE

A therapist sought a consultation in a case where he felt he had alienated a wife. He felt especially close to the husband. During a discussion of multigenerational involvement with outside systems, the husband, father of two teenage children, a boy and a girl, described how his father and paternal grandfather had been involved with outside helpers for problems with alcohol. Presently, this man and his 16-year-old son were involved with two larger systems, focusing on their problems and alcohol abuse. None of the women in the family engaged with helpers. None of the men, over the generations, had overcome their problems with alcohol. The husband stated that he had grown up hearing about the various helpers in his family's life and that his ideas about helpers were that they were warm and supportive and patient and far more understanding than wives. Indeed, as the wives showed less understanding, the helpers seemed to show more. Triadic marriages composed of husbands with alcohol problems, "understanding" helpers, and "not-so-understanding" wives existed for three generations, with no change in pattern or symptom.

Just as families have "rules" regarding interaction within the family, so do they have "rules" regarding interaction with larger systems. Such rules may have a profound effect on the entry of larger systems into a family's sphere.

One very common rule holds that most interaction with outsiders is bad and that what goes on in the family is nobody else's business. Such a rule, often unspoken to the outside systems, is certain to make the entry of larger systems very problematic and often leads to an escalating pattern of pursuit and distance between the outsiders and the family, culminating in outsiders designating the family resistant, secretive, or uncooperative and the family designating the larger systems as meddling or troublemaking.

BRIEF EXAMPLE: DON'T TALK TO OUTSIDERS ABOUT FAMILY BUSINESS

A two-parent family with an 8-year-old son and an infant girl was sent to family therapy by the son's school because the boy had been acting very babyish for several months and had become eneuretic in the classroom. Prior to the therapy referral, the boy had been sent to the school psychologist for assessment. Since the boy knew the family rule about not talking to outsiders about "family business," he refused to answer the psychologist's questions about his family, prompting the professional to assume that the boy was hiding something. When the family came for therapy, they were very confused and appeared extremely reticent. Only when the therapist began to inquire about their experience with helping professionals did it become apparent that this family had a rule against discussing problems with "strangers," and that this rule existed in both the husband's and the wife's family. At this juncture, the therapist was able to effectively pull back and respectfully place in the family's hands a decision regarding this rule. (The resolution of this case is discussed in Chapter 5 in the section "Engagement Rituals.") Without such an understanding, it would have been very easy to replicate the school psychologist's position vis-à-vis the family and fall in sync with the family's ideas about "interfering" outsiders.

In some families, the rules about outsiders are even more complex, as the mother may come from a family where the rule was "don't talk to outsiders," while the father may come from a family where the rule was "take your problems to outsiders." Without cognizance of this, helpers can be drawn into murky triangles from the moment of entering the family sphere. In this instance, where outsiders would be welcomed by the father and eschewed by the mother, it is easy to fall into unplanned alliances and splits, viewing the father as cooperative and the mother as uncooperative.

BRIEF EXAMPLE: ALTERING IATROGENIC MARITAL CONFLICT

A Chinese mother and a Caucasian father engaged with multiple helpers in a serial fashion, due to behavior problems in their 10-year-old son. The father had similar problems as a boy and felt that his family's involvement with outside systems, including school guidance counselors and scouts, had saved him from turning out "bad." The mother came from a family where children were obedient to their parents, where any problems that did arise were handled by grandparents, and where to talk to outsiders was a sign of shame. While she obeyed her husband's decision to seek outside help because she believed she must be a "good wife," she was, at the same time, terrified that her parents would find out that she was seeing a counselor and so kept this a secret from them. Her tension, the source of which was unknown to the counselor, permeated her interactions with him, leading him to label her as anxious and likely a large contributing cause in her son's misbehavior. Further, she felt unable to cooperate in tasks assigned by the counselor, while her husband gladly carried them out, leading to speculations of marital conflict as another source of the boy's problem. The present marital conflict was, in fact, iatrogenic, as the interaction with an outside system, operating from Western values, exacerbated an already difficult cross-cultural situation.

During the consultation when this profound difference in the meaning of outside help to each one's family of origin was discovered, the husband and wife commented that they had not known how important this difference was. The husband had felt that his wife was simply being stubborn and uncooperative, while the wife had thought that her husband was being disrespectful. The wife did think counseling could be useful to them but explained that she felt enormously disloyal to her family at every session. She also felt unable to tell her parents about having problems with the son, because of her fears regarding their views about going to outsiders. Consequently, the family was cut off from a possible source of support and advice, and the current family pattern vis-à-vis outsiders was skewed to the style of the husband's family of origin. During the session, the husband was shocked to realize the repetitious pattern regarding a child's behavior and outside help. Ultimately, the consultant was able to challenge the couple to develop a third alternative that did not totally replicate either family of origin but represented what they wanted for their own family regarding relationships to the outside world. The counselor, who was now able to appreciate the wife's dilemma, ceased struggling with her and became an effective coach, as both husband and wife began examining rules from their families of origin about outside help.

Many families have rules regarding particular larger systems. For instance, the rule may be that anyone who goes to a mental health center is "crazy" but talking your problems over with a priest, a rabbi, or a school counselor is acceptable. Other families may have rules against school systems, dating from the parents' youth, while regarding probation, for instance, as an appropriate rite of passage because the father and his father were on probation as teenagers.

Determinations of such rules can inform referral choices, entry decisions, and larger program development decisions. Discussion with families about such rules can increase their choices about effective engagement with larger systems.

Some families have unspoken gender rules regarding who can receive help and who can provide help. In many families in our culture only females are allowed to ask for and receive outside help. For males to do so is seen as a sign of weakness. In certain families, outside help can only be accepted if it is provided by a woman. In other families, outside help can only be accepted if it is provided by a man.

Often families are cut off from key members. Such cutoffs may be due to difficult relationships, including intense conflict between parents and adult children, conflict among grown siblings, and divorce, or they may be due to economic and political factors requiring foreign immigration or employment moves from one end of the country to another. In cutoffs both the family's familiar way to solve problems and their attitudes towards help by missing members become important. Many families engage with larger systems in order to fill the void left by the family's natural helper. If the family always turned to Aunt Margaret for help and her help was generally quite useful, but she is back in England while the family is in New York, the family, with no prior experience with helpers, may begin to turn to outside systems. Two very different circumstances will then ensue, depending on whether the family believes Aunt Margaret would approve or disapprove of their move to get outside help. If Aunt Margaret would approve, then, given no other major constraints, the helping effort will likely go well. If Aunt Margaret would disapprove, and particularly if she would feel betrayed, then it is not unusual to see a family go from one helper to another in an impossible "search for Aunt Margaret."

An often more ferocious pattern ensues when the cutoff results from divorce. It is especially important to discern the absent parent's view of professional help, since children will be sensitive and often loyal to this point of view. Thus, if a single mother is attempting to get help for herself and her children, which the children believe their father would disapprove of, the helping effort may fail.

Messages to single parents from the wider culture often imply that the family is lacking, has deficits, or is otherwise marred, justifying the enlistment of more and more helpers. It is common to see efforts by larger systems to replace a "missing" parent with helpers. Since helpers are not family members, such an effort is doomed to failure. (See the No-Exits section below for a discussion of the particular difficulties that arise when both the family and the helpers share this deficit view.)

BRIEF EXAMPLE: CUTOFFS IN THE FAMILY AND IN THE LARGER SYSTEMS

A single-parent family consisted of a mother and three daughters. The father had remarried and moved away and had maintained no contact with his former wife and children. However, his father and mother had had intense involvement with the family, serving as foster parents for the three girls during a time when both parents were in jail for selling drugs. The mother began to work very hard on rehabilitation and sought and received custody of her three children. The paternal grandparents, however, continued to want the girls' custody, and a ferocious battle ensued. The mother and the grandparents ultimately cut off from each other and refused to speak to each other. Each side then began to enlist outside helpers, characterizing the other side as bad, intractable, unworkable, and so on. Mistrust among the helpers ran extremely high, replicating the pattern in the family. Over 6 months of such engagement with helpers, one daughter, 14, moved back to the grandparents and refused contact with her mother; one daughter, 16, moved out on her own; and one daughter, 12, remained with the mother. Likewise, the pattern among the helpers involved two helpers moving firmly to the mother's side, one helper moving to the grandparents' side, and two helpers totally withdrawing. Clearly, the family pattern of cutoffs, which had deteriorated into fierce loyalty binds and the choice of "you're either for me, against me, or totally out," had been replicated in the family–helper systems.

Cutoffs in poor families, while complex, are often precipitated and/ or supported by involvement with larger systems that is required for economic survival. Welfare regulations frequently split families, while doing nothing to rebuild the family's economic viability. Homeless families that do not conform to legal definitions of marriage are often not allowed in family shelters unless the husband leaves the family. Not surprisingly, the relationships between such families and the larger systems are often conflictual, as larger system regulations serve to undermine family cohesion. Blame for the conflict is usually placed inside the family by the larger systems, and wider policy issues that operate to split families and maintain poverty remain unexamined and largely covert.

Some families become involved with many outsiders in an effort to divert attention from internal family strife that is unacceptable, unmanageable, and covert. The complex juggling of relationships with several professionals comes to consume the family's focus. Often a family with little or no prior experience with helping systems will suddenly and rapidly engage several outsiders. Frequently, in these circumstances the family will not inform one helper about the entry of other helpers.

BRIEF EXAMPLE: A FAMILY UNITES AGAINST A COMMON ENEMY

A family consisting of two parents and two teenage sons had no prior experience with helping professionals. The parents were both highly educated and highly placed in their community, and the family was one that would be expected to turn to private resources, rather than public-sector systems, when help was needed. However, following the family's return from an unsatisfactory sabbatical for the father, each parent began to enlist a host of public-sector helpers, including probation, outreach family therapy (generally reserved for "poor and disorganized families"), and an advocate for school problems, citing the son's bad behavior in the home, school, and community as the rationale. No presentation was made of any conflict between the parents, although each was rounding up outsiders separately. In fact, the parents were on the verge of divorce. This impending family breakup was kept secret from both their sons and outside helpers and became open knowledge only at a later consultation interview focusing on the family and larger systems. The boys, formerly "model" children and students, had become very stubborn at home and were refusing to obey rules at school. No actual laws had been broken, but the parents were able to convince the probation department that their sons were "at risk." As these various public-sector systems entered, they began to send family members for various assessments with psychologists, psychiatrists, and pediatricians. The family responded with hostility to these professionals, who wrote very negative reports about the family.

Within 4 months, 17 professionals became involved with the family. Strikingly, the outsiders were intensely split. Several saw the family quite favorably, and several negatively. Perhaps of more salient interest was the family's perception that all conflicts among them, including marital and parent–child, were now over, as the family united against the "hostile" helpers and in support of the "positive" helpers. Only when the various outsiders began to pull back and the family recycled their earlier interactions did the place of outside systems in promoting pseudostability become apparent.

In some families the engagement with outside systems comes to serve the function of supporting family myths that might otherwise break down. Such myths, arising in earlier family interaction, come to require larger systems for their continuance. Required family change and development is thereby obviated.

BRIEF EXAMPLE: A KNIGHT IN SHINING ARMOR

A blended family consisted of mother, stepfather, the mother's 10-year-old son from a previous marriage, and a 6-year-old daughter from the present marriage. The mother's first marriage had been extremely troubled, and she had been first abused and then abandoned by her husband. Left on her own with a young son and having little money, she met and married a man whom she considered to be her "knight in shining armor." The whole family strongly believed in the idea that it was the father's role to "save" the mother and that this savior job needed to be repeatedly assumed, thus necessitating factors in the life of the family that would ensure this process. Additionally, the stepfather had a very difficult time accepting that his wife had been married before and showed this primarily through troubled interactions with his stepson. Gradually the boy became the intense focus of family concern, and the family, at the stepfather's suggestion, began to serially enlist outside helpers, including physicians, a chiropractor, psychologists, social workers, police officers to lecture the boy, and a junior army group to provide "discipline." At a consultation devoted to eliciting the family's history with larger systems, it was discovered that as each effort, initiated by the stepfather, was tried, the mother would become very excited, feeling the answer to her son's problems had been found, while the stepfather would express subtle skepticism. Each effort would initially succeed, at which point the stepfather would begin to show signs of depression and withdraw from his wife and family. At that juncture, the son would misbehave, the wife would have her hopes dashed, and the stepfather would reemerge to support his wife during her unhappiness, thus replicating his initial entry into the system as mother's knight in shining armor. The stepfather would then enlist a different sort of helper, and the process would begin again.

Specific family patterns and themes, both nuclear and multigenerational, may profoundly affect family interaction with larger systems. Often such patterns and themes are outside of awareness and become apparent only when one begins to investigate the arena of family–larger system interaction.

LARGER SYSTEM PATTERNS AND THEMES AFFECTING ENTRY

A major factor affecting engagement of families and larger systems can be found in the wider context of giving and receiving help in our culture. Most larger systems are embedded in a deficit perspective that posits that the presence of a problem implies weakness, pathology, and often the presence of other problems. This deficit perspective informs the work of many human service systems and can readily be heard at case conferences from which workers emerge depressed and overwhelmed. Broad generalizations, frequently made about categories of people, bypass strengths and resources and focus on "deficits." For example, single-parent families are generally examined for what's missing, that is, a second adult, rather than for the strengths emergent in the family organization. Such families are generally thought to have more problems, requiring more helpers (e.g., therapy, Big Brothers, assertiveness training, etc.), when in fact, more finances and the mobilization of the family's own resources may be all the help that is needed. Families with handicapped members are more often criticized for the handling of their handicapped children than affirmed for their perseverance. It is not unusual for families to experience professionals who assume the parents could be "better parents," particularly if the family is poor and less formally educated. Such a deficit perspective profoundly affects any family's entry into interaction with larger systems, contributing to the family's response and shaping the family's sense of its own capacities.

It is important to note that a deficit view often informs preservice and in-service training designs, supervision, and evaluation of job performance within human services. Human service workers often find that they are criticized more than they are affirmed. Thus it should come as no surprise when this perspective in turn permeates work with clients.

The deficit perspective leads easily to a felt need for specialization that identifies a specific kind of helper for every aspect of a problem situation (e.g., legal, medical, therapeutic, therapeutic subspecialities, etc.). Here the multiple-helper phenomenon begins to be understandable, not simply from the family's side, as discussed above, but from the service-provider side, where the norm is to identify more and more specific problems and more and more specific outsiders. Often the definition of what it means to do a good job for a probation officer or a welfare worker is to thoroughly identify every possible problem for which there might be specialized services and then to see that referrals are made.

BRIEF EXAMPLE: IF ONE HELPER IS GOOD, MORE MUST BE BETTER

A probation officer was assigned to a 16-year-old girl with minor delinquency problems. Within 2 months, the girl and her family were sent for family therapy, marital therapy, and individual psychological assessments. The individual psychologist then promoted individual therapy for the father and began to see him. The girl got drunk on a few occasions, was labeled as alcoholic, and was sent by the probation officer to a 2-week alcohol detoxification program. By the end of 3 months the family of five had as many helpers as family members, each working in a specialized area, with little progress and much fragmentation. At this juncture when the family and helpers were seen together, the probation officer was considering referring the girl to another specialist for a "sexual assessment."

Inherent in the specialization phenomenon is the fact that each speciality speaks its own language (e.g., medical, legal, psychological, etc.), often promoting fragmentation for family and helpers alike. Individuals in a single case may be simultaneously defined as mad, bad, sick, and loyal by four different specialists. Efforts of various specialists to talk with each other and create shared meaning are often fraught with misunderstanding.

The fact of specialization is one that is not likely to change markedly in the foreseeable future. Rather, as new problems get identified, new and specialized programs emerge. The family therapist working with families and larger systems requires a fund of knowledge regarding the points of view and the language of various specialities, as well as skills to enhance clear boundaries among the specialists, who frequently tend to be either highly disengaged and unaware of each other's working premises or inappropriately working in each other's spheres, promoting a family's confusion about whom to ask for help.

Mandate and Mystifications

An often overlooked aspect of larger system engagement with families is the broad and specific mandates of the various human services. Such mandates are both overt and covert.

On a broad level, larger systems define themselves and are defined by society as care givers for the wider culture. This broad mandate informs the work of hospitals, clinics, schools, welfare, probation, and various specialized larger systems such as services for the handicapped, geriatric services, residential programs, Big Brothers and Big Sisters, and so on.

This care-giver mandate is often further refined by larger systems. Some larger systems see their job as providing people with support, protection, aid, and solving problems *for* the client, while others see their job as facilitating a person's growth and development, which generates new options and problem-solving capacities.

A second broad mandate of many of these same systems, also anticipated by the society at large, is social control. Probation, welfare, residential programs, and certain services for the handicapped and elderly are expected to constrain behavior, protect others, and, if necessary, enforce specific limitations, such as when people may see each other, for how long, and under what circumstances; how people must spend their time (e.g., one *must* attend a certain class or number of group therapy sessions); where people may live (e.g., residential programs); or how people may spend their money (e.g., discretionary fund mandates for handicapped adults).

Frequently the care-giver mandate and the social-control mandate exist in a profound tension within the larger system, generating confusion and mystification for workers and families alike. The purposes of initial engagement are often murky or shift rapidly from one mandate to the other without clarification. Thus, a person on probation may be "counseled" by his probation officer within a care-giving frame, but the sharing of certain information may immediately generate a social-control relationship. A family may be sent by a welfare worker to therapy and find that the definitions of therapy, as a generative process, and social control, as a constraining process, are blurred for all concerned.

Various larger systems also have specific mandates to work in certain ways with particular populations. Generally, specific mandates are inextricably bound to funding streams and current social trends. For example, in the 1960s it was possible to receive federal grants to train encounter-group leaders, while in the early 1970s it was fairly easy to receive funding for drug abuse prevention and treatment programs. In the earlier 1980s it was far easier to receive funding for eating disorders than it was for drug abuse. In 1987 a renewed interest in drug abuse has widened that funding stream; however, it would no doubt be impossible to receive funding for encounter groups. The sources of such funding affect system mandates, as can be seen in an examination of the larger systems that emerged to deal with drug abuse and were funded by the

U.S. Justice Department versus those funded by the National Institute of Mental Health. The former systems were far more interested in social control, while the latter generally worked in the care-giving and generative arena. Often the funding underpinning of specific mandates is ignored by larger systems or treated as a "necessary evil" and is unknown to families, thus becoming a source of mystification affecting the process of engagement between families and larger systems.

The beliefs that shape specific mandates deeply affect family–larger system involvement. If a larger system mandate to work with a certain population is informed by the belief that a problem is chronic, unsolvable, or manageable, but lifelong, this will set a family and the larger system on a very different course of action than if the belief is that a problem is an opportunity or a normative developmental crisis.

The larger system organized as "Big Brother–Big Sister" or "Uncles and Aunts at Large" is a good example. Its specific mandate is to work with individual children from single-parent families. The parent, usually the mother, is advised, indeed ordered, to remain at a distance from this Big Brother–little brother relationship. The often unspoken belief underpinning this specific mandate is that such children are lacking a "role model." For boys a Big Brother or "Uncle" is assigned, with the implicit message from the larger system to the family that the boy will not grow up "normally" without a male role model. An even more denigrating message is sent when the child is a girl living with her mother and is seen to need a Big Sister. Clearly the belief underpinning the mandate is that single parents, left to their own devices, will lessen a child's chance for healthy psychological development. Rarely is an attempt made to investigate the natural resources of the single-parent family (Morawetz & Walker, 1984).

Beliefs in the larger system, and consequently the messages to clients, may be contradictory. For instance, a larger system designed to work with mentally handicapped adults may operate by the simultaneous and mutually incompatible beliefs of lifelong handicap and complete normalization.

The beliefs underpinning specific mandates often support the continued existence of the problem requiring larger system involvement in the first place.

BRIEF EXAMPLE: FROM HOPE TO HOPELESSNESS

A family was sent for therapy by their family physician upon the discovery of bulimic symptoms in a 17-year-old daughter. The girl had had such symptoms for about a year but had kept this secret. The family was naive regarding larger helping systems. They appeared very distraught and eager to seek help. They left the first session quite hopeful that action would ensue and were determined to do their part. Between the first and second session, the mother, who was understandably frantic to get all manner of help for her daughter, saw an ad for a lecture on anorexia and bulimia, sponsored by a larger system whose specific and self-appointed mandate was to work with "eating disorders." For $20 each the mother and daughter went to a 1-hour lecture. The family returned for the second session and appeared full of despair, for they had "learned" that the girl *had bulimia*, that this would pervade every aspect of her life, that "bulimia was incurable," and that she would need all manner of therapy (individual, group, and family) just to cope.

The broad and specific mandates of larger systems are often put in place at a point in history and then remain unexamined or unquestioned. They become part of the untouchable mythology of an agency or program, such that while actual services may change over time, the original mandate lurks in the background, affecting current services. Thus it is not unusual to find, upon detailed enquiry, that a place offering marriage and family therapy was formerly a guidance clinic whose mandate was to see mothers and children separately, never to see fathers, and to "save" children from these mothers, or that a child residential service was formerly a home for "unwed mothers," and before that was a foundling home for poor orphans.

Unexamined mandates create a soft hum in the background of larger systems, effecting a mystification of purpose.

BRIEF EXAMPLE: SHIFTING MANDATES

A children's residential program, publicly funded, had emerged out of a church-related institution devoted to housing orphans and providing care for poor and poorly educated unwed mothers, while counseling them to give their babies up for adoption. This earlier mandate was an accurate reflection of predominant social views existing from 1930, when the system began, to 1965, when services for orphans and unwed mothers ended, and services for "emotionally disturbed" children began. Church influence remained during and after this transition. Families of the children in residence began to be seen in therapy; however, the families and children were seen within the context of the prior and now covert mandate, which stipulated that they were objects of pity and charity, while the more current and overt mandate was to facilitate their growth and development. The clash of these obviously contradictory mandates made work between the families and the larger systems fraught with confusing messages and mystifying expectations.

Social Policy: Norms, Shifts, and Crises

Larger systems exist within a context of social policy, political decision making, and laws that shape and direct their work. These rise out of the socioeconomic context of the culture.

For the larger systems engaging with families, this factor is especially salient, as the social policy regarding families in North America continues to reflect traditional values and promote the nuclear family form of two parents, two children, father employed outside the home, and mother remaining at home, a family form that represents only 10% of current families (Pogrebin, 1983). Unexamined in any critical way, such social policy informs larger system beliefs and actions such that families that deviate from the so-called traditional family are often viewed as aberrant and problem-filled or problem-inducing (e.g., single-parent families, stepparent families, families where women work outside the home, etc.).

Social policy regarding families in North America is exemplified in the lack of adequate child care, the high infant mortality rate among the poor, reflecting inadequate larger systems for health care delivery, welfare regulations that split families, housing policies that underpin and support a growing homeless population, lack of paid maternity leave, and so on. What is especially confounding is that such social policy exists within a rhetoric that idealizes families, thus mystifying families and larger systems alike. Our larger systems spring from social policy norms that at one and the same time venerate mythical families and denigrate the integrity of actual families.

Such social policy also reflects the culture's view towards minorities, in turn affecting larger systems' work with minority families. For instance, for many years in the United States, the Moynihan report (Moynihan, 1965) on black families informed the work of many larger systems engaged with black families. This report postulated weaknesses and deficits in the black family, using white, middle-class values as the measuring stick. Blame for such problems as poverty and crime were placed on the black family structure in a classic victim-blaming scheme. Such a viewpoint neatly shifted responsibilities from the larger social structure, underpinned by centuries of racist economics and politics, to the smaller family structure. Any focus on strengths inherent in this family structure was missing, and only pathology was postulated. While subsequently challenged by black researchers and family sociologists (Webb-Woodward, 1980), the thinking in this report still informs many larger systems who work with black families. A similar phenomenon can be seen in Canada regarding the Native American population, for whom social policy and law has been developed by white and upper-middle-class policy makers. Adoption and foster placement systems have routinely removed Native American children from their homes and extended kinship systems and sent them hundreds or even thousands of miles away to white families. Such a policy obviously implies that the Native American family form is seen as weaker, less advantageous, deficit ridden, and so on. Programs and funding options that would respect the natural ecology of this population are ignored in favor of those that in fact promote further erosion of strengths. Most recently, attempts by Native American social workers to be involved in policy shaping for welfare programs for their own communities have been rebuffed. Such decisions profoundly effect the shape of larger systems who interact with families, promulgating a view of the "correct" family.

Larger systems must deal with frequent shifts in social policy, placing demands on their organizations. The rationale for the shift is often unclear and training for it nonexistent. Confusion and anger in workers often cascade to their interactions with families.

A recent example can be seen in the social policy shift to deinstitutionalization of the mentally ill and mentally handicapped (MacKinnon & Marlett, 1984). Vast numbers of larger systems scaled down and retooled, while many new systems sprang up, often with little training and inadequate funding. Communities where group homes were to be placed were often ill-prepared. Families who learned to believe one point of view about their handicapped member were being told they must now accept another point of view, with little preparation or plans for working with the stress thus induced. Escalating misunderstandings between families and larger systems often ensued.

A similar example is the shift to provide special education services within public schools, often with initial inadequate preparation and training for school personnel. Such lack of training led easily to feelings of incompetence, then of anger, and finally of blame placing, usually on the children and their families, since they were available while the policy makers were not. In both of these examples, it is important to note that the specific content of the social policy shifts, that is, deinstitutionalization and integration, were humane, appropriate, and necessary, but that by ignoring the process and the impact on frontline workers whose job it is to carry out policy shifts, the net effect is to engender an increased sense of disempowerment, which cascades through the ecosystem, often negatively affecting the interaction between larger systems and family members and maintaining the status quo, regardless of the new content (Bell, 1982; Sarason & Doris, 1979).

Sometimes social policy shifts dramatically, albeit temporarily, in response to local crises that, in turn, affect the day-to-day operations of larger systems and their interactions with families. Examples of crises include the child-abuse murder of foster children and the committing of a violent act by a group home resident. The interplay of law, the media, and public opinion converge, often reducing enormous complexity to a scapegoating process. What might effectively be viewed as a symptom of dysfunction in the wider social context, leading to effective policy shifts with concomitant shifts in training and supervision, is, rather, localized, with blame placed on individual workers.

Commissions are appointed, studies are made, evidence of incompetence is gathered, memos are sent, and often an atmosphere of fear, timidity, uncertainty, and greater social control is generated in frontline workers, who communicate this in turn to their clients.

BRIEF EXAMPLE: CRISIS CONTAGION

A family–larger system consultation was sought by a family therapist who felt that his work was stymied by increasing social-control actions in the other larger systems, welfare and probation. Indeed, as he began to present the case, there appeared to be control placed on the identified patient, a 16-year-old boy, who had unsubstantiated charges pending against him for verbally harassing a girl on the school bus. The boy, who had a record of petty crimes, had been removed from his home and placed in a locked facility, and was awaiting trial. When the consultation was arranged, the therapist was told by the residential program that he would need a court order for the boy to attend. Such an order was issued, stating that the boy must wear handcuffs, traveling to and during the interview, despite the fact that no history of violence was alleged. The unexplainable order and the increasing elements of social control began to make a degree of sense when participants in the presession told the consultant that another teenage girl had recently been murdered by a different boy in the same community, while this boy had been on a pass from the residential treatment center. This crisis formed a major part of the current context and informed the actions of the larger systems.

Examination of a helping context in which a recent crisis has occurred may uncover a larger system's sense of dependence on an uncertain sociopolitical climate, resulting in apathy, cynicism, and despair in those workers whose very job it is to ameliorate apathy, cynicism, and despair in clients.

Leadership and Staffing Patterns in Larger Systems

Changes in leadership in larger systems occur fairly frequently, often with attendant periods of upheaval. At the local level, staffs must deal with changes in style of leadership, loyalty issues vis-à-vis prior leaders, questions of attachment in a rapidly changing environment, and a backdrop of anxiety regarding one's own position. Because of frequent turnover, one's peer often becomes one's supervisor in a short time span.

Changes in leadership may or may not be accompanied by alterations in specific practices. It is not unusual for unrealizable hopes to be placed on a new human service system leader, who must struggle with identical constraints as the prior leader and may be unable to alter practices. Frontline workers who have been through many leadership changes often come to view any new leader with skepticism or pessimism, thus contributing to stasis. Conversations with many larger system workers yield only slight variations of "I just do my job. He or she isn't going to be able to really change anything around here. I've seen it all before." Such cynicism becomes an element in the family–larger system context.

Workers in larger systems are often initially drawn to their work by a desire to help others, to work with people, and to participate in enhancing life for particular population groups. Many larger systems utilize paraprofessionals or very recent graduates, frequently placing them in positions for which they have little or no prior practical training and giving them limited and usually administrative, rather than clinical, supervision. They are expected to do the difficult work of assessment, intervention, and rehabilitation with various populations, who have often been *defined by others* as being in need of services. Thus, the stage is often set for problematic interaction between uncertain or insecure workers and frightened or angry clients.

EXITS

Many families engage with larger systems for a specified period of time and complete work to the satisfaction of all concerned. The family reports feeling pleased with itself. Subsequent engagements by such families with larger systems are colored by a tone of optimism based on prior experience.

Other families leave specific larger systems because of dissatisfaction with services offered. Such families are not coerced or ordered to engage with helpers and often have a sense of their rights as consumers of a service. Their dissatisfaction may influence any subsequent engagement with larger systems, but such families are often able to raise this problem early on and clarify their expectations with any new helper. It is crucial at this juncture that the family's viewpoint regarding prior dissatisfaction be listened to carefully and not dismissed as growling, for in understanding such dissatisfaction may lie the seeds of a new and more successful engagement.

Families may exit from one larger system via referral to another larger system. The referral process in larger systems has a powerful impact on the course of involvement between families and outsiders and on whether or not a family acquires multiple helpers. The act of a referral is embedded in the specific nature of the relationship between the family and the referral source (Selvini Palazzoli *et al.*, 1980).

If the family and the referring person are quite close and comfortable with one another, then referral may be experienced by the family as very confusing or as an act of rejection. This may pose engagement and subsequent exit difficulties with the new helper.

BRIEF EXAMPLE: LOYALTY TO THE REFERRING PERSON

A family consisting of a widowed mother, a 14-year-old son, Keith, and a 12-year-old daughter, Ann, were referred for family therapy by the son's probation officer. The family had experienced severe turmoil, beginning with the son's delinquent behavior of 1 year's duration and culminating in the tragic suicide by gunshot of the father, 3 months before the referral. The father blamed his suicide on his son, leaving a note stating that the son's behavior caused his death. The probation officer had been positively engaged with the son and the mother before the father's death. In vain, she had tried to engage the father as well.

Following his death, she gave a great deal of appropriate support to the family. Unknown to the family, however, she was suffering enormous guilt for not realizing the extent of the father's anguish in life, and her supervisor believed she needed to refer the family to a therapist. She did so but was unable to explain her reasons for the referral. The family, however, sensed her discomfort and pain and, out of loyalty to her prior support of them, refused to engage actively with the therapist. They would go to sessions and sit quietly, answering politely and minimally when the therapist asked questions. The boy continued to see the probation officer individually and continually asked her to see his mother again. Finally, at a family–larger system interview held with all concerned, the confusion surrounding the referral process became clear, as did the boy's plan to commit another petty crime in order to keep the probation officer in the family sphere.

If, on the other hand, the family and the referral source are not on good terms, the referral may be tainted with anger and frustration. The family may experience the referral for specific services as a sign of blame. This is especially true when referrals are made for family therapy without adequate explanation of what such work is or with a tone that emphasizes *family* as the locus of the problem.

Referral may signify the exit of one larger system from the family sphere and the entrance of another, or it may signify an additive process in which a new helper is added while the prior one remains, expects frequent and detailed reports, sets the agenda for the new work, and is, in fact, part of the system to be considered. This occurs most often, although not exclusively, when families are coerced to go for help.

Some families and larger systems disengage with one another through a process of reciprocal apathy. A family may repeatedly break appointments or simply not show up. Rather than actively discovering the reasons for not showing up, the larger system worker, who is often overburdened with too big a caseload, may wait to hear from the family, interpreting the broken appointment as lack of interest. The family, in turn, interprets not hearing from the worker as lack of interest, and disengagement ensues.

NO-EXITS

Some families and larger systems exist in seemingly never-ending interaction with one another. Often, specific families become known within a network of larger systems, and if asked, neither the family nor the helpers can envision a future without one another, even if this involvement is negative and unpleasant. The family and helpers may agree on one unsolvable problem, eschewing emergent solutions because they do not fit some preconceived idea about the problem and possible solutions. Or as each particular problem is solved, new problems may be identified, requiring the maintenance of larger systems in the family sphere. Family interaction with larger systems regarding a deficit view of family functioning, disparate ideas regarding mandates both between family and larger systems and among larger systems, and multigenerational legacies regarding helpers all contribute to the no-exit phenomenon.

Many families readily accept the same deficit view of family functioning that pervades the larger systems. This view is popularized in the media; one can rarely pick up a popular magazine without finding an article on the "delaying family," the "betraying family," or the "decaying family." Many parents' confidence in their parenting styles, their marital interaction, their sexual relationship, or their children's development has eroded and been replaced by a pervasive sense of wrongdoing. Families whose organization reflects a form varying from the two-parent nuclear family exist in a wider context that defines them as deficit ridden. When the family and the larger system share this deficit view, it becomes difficult to know when outside help should cease. Often the family and the outside helpers like each other and settle in to a long-lasting cycle of perceived need and provision of help, which discovers the next perceived need.

BRIEF EXAMPLE: AN ESCALATING SENSE OF DEFICITS

A single-parent mother, divorced 3 years, lived with her teenage daughter. The mother had had a number of disappointing relationships with men, and although she worked outside the home and provided for her family, she viewed herself and her family unit as filled with deficits. Her parents believed a single mother could not succeed, as did most of her friends. In short, she was embedded in a context that viewed her and her family as lacking, rather than resourceful. Since she felt quite unhappy, she initiated a counseling relationship. At this juncture, her daughter, likely responding to her mother's sadness and testing her own independence, began to misbehave, first refusing to keep a curfew and escalating with more provocative behavior, such as misusing alcohol and staying out over night. The counselor referred the mother to social services, who recommended removing the girl and placing her in a foster home, clearly delineating the mother as unable to cope as a single parent. She agreed with this view and signed a custody-by-agreement contract to last 6 months and then be reviewed. During the 6 months, the girl continued to misbehave, insisting that she wanted to go home. The foster parents blamed this on the mother and complained that visits home were disruptive. The mother agreed and visits were sharply curtailed, resulting in further misbehavior by the girl, who stated that she felt rejected. The mother believed, however, that the foster home could give her daughter much more than she could, because there were two parents, other children, and adequate finances to go on nice outings. Social services concurred with this view and cited the mother's unfortunate choices in men as evidence to keep the girl out. Mother and daughter were framed as jealous of one another, and while there was no evidence to support this view, the mother began to worry that this might be true. After 6 months, the girl's foster placement was continued, no work was initiated towards reunification, and the mother grew less and less sure of herself. During the second 6 months, the mother was involved in a serious car accident, in which she was hit from the rear. Both she and those helping her psychologized about the "meaning" of the accident, and a view grew that she needed even more help, leading to the placement in her home of a homemaker aide for 10 hours a day, whose primary job was to talk to the mother and keep her from being too lonely. At a family–larger system interview, attended by the mother and six professionals and paraprofessionals representing mental health, social services, education, and foster care, it became apparent that the mother and the helpers were all in agreement regarding her "deficits," that no one had a view of her strengths, and that eventual disengagement was in no one's future scenario.

Some families and larger systems have difficulty disengaging because the larger systems have put services in place that confirm a view of deficits, which the family grudgingly, or sometimes shamefully, accepts while communicating resentment towards the helpers, which becomes further confirmation of the family's lack of resources. Often the larger systems provide that which the family cannot afford for their children, as when children go into foster homes and are given more expensive clothing or diet or when Big Brothers or Big Sisters take children on outings that the parents are not allowed to join and cannot financially manage on their own. Here a cycle emerges in which the family experiences itself as less and less able to provide, more and more out of touch with its own natural resources, and permanently dependent on larger systems.

At times, families respond with anger towards a deficit view of their functioning. Such anger is often underpinned by fear regarding the power of larger systems. If, however, the family is not knowledgeable about strategies for interacting with larger systems, such anger will again be seen as confirmation of deficits, and the family may find itself coerced to interact with larger systems in a spiraling cycle of mutual anger and blame.

BRIEF EXAMPLE: IGNORING A FAMILY'S STRENGTHS

A family moved to Canada from Chile in order to escape political persecution. Their prior experiences with larger systems was that they were agents of an oppressive government. Further, they viewed their family as strong and had well-established problem-solving methods that depended on parental authority. The move to Canada, involving the likelihood that they would never return to Chile, put a lot of stress on family members. For the first time ever, the father was unemployed and the mother was working outside the home. The family was cut off from natural supports, knew little English, and was suffering economically. A 12-year-old daughter, the oldest of the three, was caught shoplifting, necessitating family interaction with police, probation, and child welfare. Family fear at the sight of police at their door was expressed by the father's loud anger towards his daughter, convincing child welfare that he was a bad parent. The welfare worker, a young woman, ordered the parents to "parenting classes" and sent the family for family therapy. The parents, especially the father, insisted their family could solve their own problems. This was taken as further evidence of his intransigence, and more helpers were added, as the children were sent for psychological assessments. The family became unable to extricate itself from larger systems, and the daughter was eventually put in a group home.

Since a deficit view of family functioning posits static, knowable norms for families and sets helpers on a course of treating families to fit those norms, changes that do not fit a predetermined view of what constitutes success may not be recognized by helpers or by families, and appropriate disengagement will not occur. In their interactions with larger systems, families often change in unexpected ways. If such changes are not acknowledged or affirmed as valid choices, then the family may find itself sent to other helpers and examined for other problems in a never-ending cycle.

A family's expectation of a larger system may be out of sync with that system's view of its own mandate, resulting in a spiraling cycle of blame, disappointment, and anger. The family may hunt for other helpers or may find itself the recipient of criticism or a bevy of referrals. For instance, a family with a child in need of special education services may expect that a school system's mandate is to provide such educational services as their child requires. The school, on the other hand, may view its mandate as much broader, including family psychological assessment and subsequent intervention. If the family views this as an intrusion, the school may then view the family as resistant, and needed educational services for the child may suffer as the family and school enter into a war with each other.

Some families find themselves caught between two or more larger systems whose mandates conflict or are in opposition. Harrell's work (1980) indicated that when larger systems conflict with one another regarding treatment of a particular family, the family often becomes part of an enduring triangle and can exist over two and three generations as part of a troubled agency–family triad.

BRIEF EXAMPLE: A CLASH OF MANDATES

A family consisting of a single-parent mother and two children in foster care was sent by their welfare worker to family therapy. The welfare worker's mandate was one of social control, and she saw her primary job as that of protecting children. The referral to family therapy was viewed by her and her supervisor as within this social-control mandate, and she expected the therapist to teach specific parenting skills, to act as a monitor for family visits that were occurring at the therapy sessions, and to send frequent reports regarding the family's "cooperation" with treatment. The family therapist viewed his mandate as generating choices for the family, and when the family indicated that their idea about family therapy was that it was to reunite them, he began to work on that. In short order, conflict emerged between the welfare worker, who felt the family was not ready for reunification and who was under pressure to make the foster placements permanent because the children had been out of their own home for a year and welfare policy required such permanent placement, and the family therapist, who felt the family should have increased time together, leading to reunification. The family members grew confused and demoralized, as each larger system enlisted other helpers to support its view. Examination of this immediate triangle yielded long-standing conflicts of this nature between the welfare system and the therapy clinic, regardless of who the specific workers were, with frequent deterioration in family coping, leading to the input of further help, and a family existence marked by more or less permanent interaction with larger systems.

Conflicting family and family-of-origin beliefs regarding the efficacy of outside help to solve a problem, a deficit view of family functioning held by family and helpers alike, the formation of family–larger system triangles, and larger system specialization all converged in the following case.

CASE EXAMPLE: A FAMILY BORN WITH LARGER SYSTEMS

A family was referred by a dietician because of the unusual eating habits of the oldest daughter. The Moore family consisted of a mother, Caroline, age 30; father, Alan, age 33; daughter, Sandra, age 12; and daughter, Ellen, age 8. The referral stated that Sandra was anorexic and that family treatment was deemed necessary (see Figure 2-1).

During the first interview, several salient issues emerged. Individual assessment of Sandra indicated that she was far from anorexic. Rather, she had unusual preferences that consisted of eating primarily french fries, bread, and milk. She was small for her age but had not experienced any significant weight loss. Her ways of eating had been a problem to the family, and particularly to her mother, since she was an infant. She was born, when Caroline was only 17, with a congenital heart problem, requiring ongoing family interaction with medical helpers. Caroline always took Sandra to the doctor and reported on these visits to Alan, who thus remained more distant from both larger systems and the anxiety generated by his daughter's heart condition. He easily fell into the role of reassurer to his wife, whose job it was to express the family's fear about Sandra's future life.

One year prior to the involvement in therapy, Sandra's heart condition had been surgically corrected. Following the attenuation of relationships between the family and physicians, Caroline decided to seek help with Sandra's eating problems.

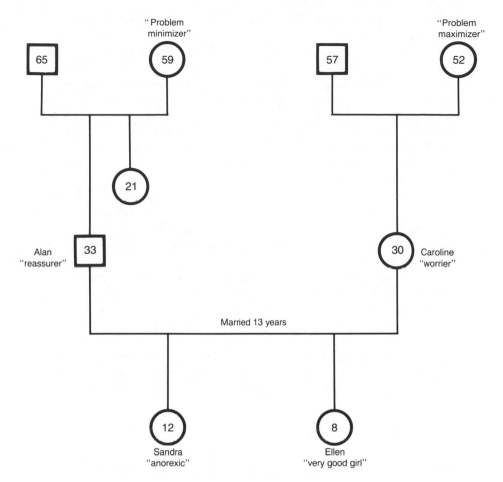

Figure 2-1. The Moore family genogram and role labels.

Her sister, Ellen, was pictured by the family as a "very good girl, who will eat anything." Several issues and patterns emerged during the interview.

1. Caroline saw the problem as huge. Alan saw the problem as more minor. All agreed that Caroline was the most worried, most upset, most concerned about the problem. A pattern of escalating complementarity between the parents prevailed.

2. Caroline and Sandra struggled daily over Sandra's eating. The struggles only occurred at dinner, the one meal when Alan was home. During other meals the girl was left alone to eat bread and milk. While Caroline and Sandra fought, Alan usually left the room and watched

television, replicating his earlier position vis-à-vis Sandra's heart condition and Caroline's involvement with her over this. A cross-generational triad, involving a covert alliance between father and daughter, was evident.

3. Caroline's mother believed the problem was severe. She was a strong believer in outside help. Caroline talked with her mother frequently about the problem, and her mother often sent her books and articles about anorexia. In prior years, she had done similarly regarding Sandra's heart problem. Conversely, Alan's mother believed the problem was minor and told her daughter-in-law to leave Sandra alone. She had been similarly distant as regards to Sandra's health. She was a private person and mistrusted professional help. Thus the struggle over definition of the problem and how to handle it, as seen in the parents, was replicated in the two sides of the extended family. The escalating complementarity of the parents' relationship was also replicated in extended-family relationships.

4. Caroline and her mother believed Sandra would stop eating altogether and would die in 2 or 3 years. Alan's mother believed Sandra would begin to eat normally on her own, in 2 or 3 years. Triadic patterns involving Sandra and the extended family were evident.

5. Sandra had a great deal of difficulty stating her own preferences in any area except food. Normal young adolescent development of ideas that differed from one's parents seemed to be either lacking or inexpressible. Sandra's difficulties in stating preferences were mirrored by her mother, who deferred to her husband and to experts.

Since the family had been referred by another professional, the dietician, it was decided to devote a portion of the interview to exploring the family's relationships with professional helpers. Several crucial factors emerged.

1. Because of Sandra's congenital heart problem the family had a long history with professionals. Indeed, there was never a time in the life of the family when professional helpers were not engaged with it. As Caroline said, "She was born with a congenital heart defect. I was 17 at the time. The doctor came in and told me the baby had a heart problem and then said 'don't worry about it'." Caroline's tone as she relayed this incident was one of frustration and near contempt. Her initial involvement with a professional left her feeling unsupported, mirroring her experience with both her husband and her father. She began to turn more and more to her mother for support and to physicians for answers.

2. According to Caroline, Sandra's eating problems developed in infancy and continued to the present. Frequently Caroline would complain to her family physician (a second professional) and ask for help.

According to Caroline, the physician's response was, "Leave her alone. She'll eat when she's hungry." Without realizing it, the physician had joined ranks with Alan and his mother, leading Caroline to redouble her efforts to make Sandra eat. The effect of the outside helper's inadvertent alliance with the father and grandmother contributed to the escalating and increasingly untenable struggle between Caroline and Sandra.

3. All direct involvements with outside helpers were the province of the mother (this is a very common situation supported by family and larger systems, easily leading to the unintentional siding cited above). Such involvement served to support the already problematic pattern of Caroline's being the lone parent concerned with Sandra's eating, and Alan's remaining aloof.

4. Following Sandra's successful recovery from serious heart surgery, Caroline decided it was time to tackle the eating problem with professional help. One may hypothesize that close involvement with outsiders had become necessary and familiar to family functioning. Rather than reorganize without professionals, the family sought a new one in the dietician.

5. The dietician believed the problem was a very serious one. Her diagnosis of anorexia in a child who would eat half a loaf of bread for lunch easily aligned her with Caroline and her mother. Alan discounted the dietician as a useful or necessary helper. Alan's mother argued with Caroline regarding the necessity of professional help. Now the professional network completely mirrored the family constellation. Caroline, her mother, and the dietician believed Sandra had a serious, life-threatening condition, in need of immediate attention. Alan, his mother, and the physician believed in backing off and that Sandra would start to eat normally in time. Each position encouraged an exacerbation of the other position. A pattern of escalating complementarity pervaded the family–professional system. As one side minimized the problem, the other side maximized the problem. The system was paralyzed. Both Caroline and Alan requested that another helper be brought in, that is, the family therapist. This request may be seen as an effort to break the deadlock, while simultaneously doing what had become familiar for the family, which was to engage with outsiders. (See Figure 2-2).

6. Exploration of the dietician's role with the family revealed that she interacted primarily with Sandra. Caroline and Sandra would go to the appointment together, but Caroline arranged for the dietician to see Sandra alone, out of the belief that Sandra would open up with her. Caroline believed, as many parents do, that the professional would be able to accomplish what she had not been able to do, namely, make Sandra eat. In point of fact, Sandra regarded the dietician with great derision, and the dietician, unknowingly, replicated Caroline's unsuccessful strategies.

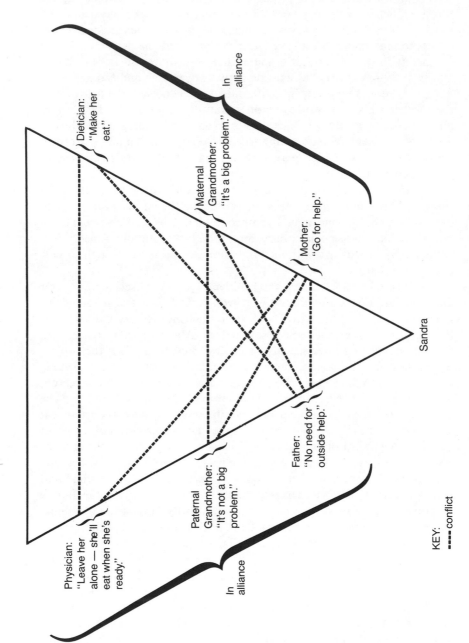

Physician: "Leave her alone — she'll eat when she's ready."

Dietician: "Make her eat."

In alliance

Maternal Grandmother: "It's a big problem."

Mother: "Go for help."

Paternal Grandmother: "It's not a big problem."

Father: "No need for outside help."

Sandra

In alliance

KEY:
▬▬ conflict

Figure 2-2. The Moore family–health care system triad.

THERAPIST: (*to mother*) What do you imagine happens when Sandra sees the dietician?

CAROLINE: I think the dietician does a lot of talking and Sandra does a lot of crying.

THERAPIST: (*to Sandra*) Is that right?

SANDRA: Well, sometimes, More often, I just listen to a lecture (*tone of contempt*).

THERAPIST: What does the dietician tell you?

SANDRA: (*with derision*) She talks a lot about kiwi fruit!

Sandra emerged each week from the dietician's office with a list of two new foods to try. She handed this to her mother, who then made a special trip to the store to purchase the items, thus involving her more in Sandra's unusual eating style. Unaware of the family's process and organization vis-à-vis Sandra's eating, the dietician's suggestions inadvertently supported the very patterns that needed to be changed. During the week, struggles would then ensue, as Caroline attempted to get Sandra to eat the new items.

THERAPIST: (*to Sandra*) Do you think getting some outside help with this problem has improved things or made the situation worse?

SANDRA: (*crying*) Worse.

THERAPIST: (*to Alan*) What do you think?

ALAN: Well, her eating hasn't changed. Frankly, I didn't think the dietician would help. Now she and her mother fight more than before seeing the dietician.

While Caroline had initiated the original contact with the dietician and while she diligently shopped for items the dietician wanted Sandra to eat, she also found it impossible to carry out the dietician's instructions. At the point of referral to family therapy, Caroline reported growing disenchantment with the dietician and was following her instructions less and less. Nonetheless, she planned for Sandra to continue her weekly visits to the dietician.

It was clear in this interview that this was a system where the potential for triangulation of the therapist was rife. The father and mother, two grandmothers, and two professionals were aligned in perfect balance. A new ally for either side would temporarily tip the balance and likely result in the search for yet another helper by whichever side felt unsupported. Also, since half the system appeared to believe that outside help was unnecessary, solutions that seemed to come from professionals ran the risk of discounting half the family.

Finally, the family had tried various "common-sense" solutions, such as the physician's advice to back off and the dietician's advice to push Sandra to eat. None of these had worked, as they too clearly mirrored the family's own struggle. The family, and Caroline in particular, felt like failures and anticipated criticism from professionals, as this had been implied in all earlier solution attempts.

This assessment of the family–multiple-helpers system led the therapist in several key directions that permeated the entire therapy.

To begin, neutrality provided the family with an unexpected relationship with a professional, one that differed from their previous notions of help. The therapist maintained a stance of openness and curiosity in the relational domain but refused to be drawn into the alliance patterns. She was careful neither to minimize the problem and thereby join Alan nor maximize it and thereby join Caroline. Neutrality had the effect of putting the parents on the same level, altering their previous complementary pattern. The therapist also maintained neutrality towards the entire notion of outside help. She did not instruct the family regarding their relationship with the dietician.

The creation of an unanticipated relationship with a professional was further enhanced by the kinds of interventions utilized. All interventions were framed as experiments or information gathering, rather than as proposed solutions. The parents were frequently encouraged to talk over and decide whether or not to do a particular experiment, thus blocking credit to the therapist for any changes that might ensue and placing ownership for the changes within the family.

The first intervention was an "odd days and even days" ritual in which the parents alternated who dealt with Sandra's eating. This intervention was based on a hypothesis that conceptualized Sandra's symptom as supporting and supported by a system whose overarching pattern was escalating complementarity. Each parent was encouraged to approach the issue in his or her unique way. Involving both parents and confirming their involvement as important implicitly introduced a symmetrical pattern to the parental dyad. This ritual had the immediate effect of engaging Alan in the therapeutic endeavor, which no outside helper had previously attempted. The therapist's neutrality towards the outcome of this ritual implicitly communicated that there would be no criticism or siding in this family–professional relationship.

A second intervention furthered the development of an unexpected relationship with an outsider, as the therapist requested that the family bring dinner to the second session. Families with eating disorder difficulties fully anticipate that the therapist will be judging their behavior vis-à-vis the meal. Instead, a relaxed atmosphere is engendered, as the therapist simply conducts the interview while all partake of the meal. Being asked to bring dinner to the clinic was unusual for the family, setting this professional endeavor apart from previous attempts. Even more unusual, however, was the total absence of advice giving. Sandra's "eating disorder" was reframed as "having favorites," altering the family map of three normal people and one anorexic and the prior helpers' map of the overinvolved mother to a map of four people with likes and dislikes, and two competent parents expanding their daughter's repertoire. This intervention operated simultaneously on the individual, family, and family-larger system levels to encourage the declaration of preferences and opinions.

Rather than framing herself as an expert, the therapist frequently adopted a one-down stance with the family, thereby framing them as the experts.

As this case proceeded, relying primarily on neutrality, rituals whose efficacy the parents were continually asked to determine, and team splits highlighting two divergent opinions and thus facilitating the parents' coming together and making explicit judgments about professional help, the parents began to insist that the therapist help them to work together as a team, Caroline decided to fire the dietician, an ally no longer necessary, and Sandra began to eat a wide variety of foods. A family "born" with larger systems, necessitated by Sandra's heart condition, had been a no-exit family for 12 years, interacting with larger systems in ways that further rigidified family patterns. The family ultimately exited from larger systems in a manner that enhanced their sense of their own resources and empowerment. (A termination ritual designed to facilitate this family's sense of its own problem-solving capacity is presented in Chapter 5.)

Appreciating the entry and exit context out of which family–larger system problems develop may, as in the foregoing case, enable the family therapist to develop new, efficacious ways of working that would not otherwise be available. The job of the family therapist becomes one of assessment at multiple levels, including individual, couple, parent–child, extended family, and family–larger system, and intervention in replicating patterns and systems of meaning throughout the macrosystem.

CHAPTER 3

Family–Larger System Assessment Model

Family–larger system assessment involves the therapist in an extra level of information-gathering and direction-setting activities. This work should enhance and augment, not replace, individual and family assessment. The macrosystemic concepts discussed in this chapter not only inform ongoing individual and family work but also establish a basis for intervention in the macrosystem.

CASE EXAMPLE: FAMILY–LARGER SYSTEM MAZE

(This case will be elaborated in segments throughout this chapter.) Two almost simultaneous referrals to family therapy were made for the same family by two social workers employed by a government social service agency. The family consisted of Mr. and Mrs. Connors, two daughters, 15 and 17, and two foster daughters, 13 and 14. The parents had had various foster children in their home for their entire 20-year marriage. Consequently, they had interacted quite regularly with many social workers from social services. Most of these foster children had emotional and social problems of varying degrees. The family had never sought family therapy before nor had they been referred for family therapy prior to the present referrals.

The two social workers who made the referrals were involved with the family as workers for each of the two foster children. Separately, both had become alarmed by behavior in the foster child for whom they were responsible and, unbeknownst to each other, referred the family for family therapy. The referrals were made to the same agency, but to two different therapists. After calls to the family this was discovered, and one therapist agreed to work with the family while the other would be behind the one-way mirror. At this juncture several weeks passed while the

44

family therapist waited to hear from the family to set an appointment. Finally, Mrs. Connors called and made the first appointment, expressing, however, that it would be very difficult to get everyone in the family together because of work and school schedules. Subsequently, the time of the first appointment was changed twice.

The family arrived and expressed a great deal of confusion about the referral for family therapy. They agreed that each foster daughter had serious problems but believed the locus of such problems was in the girls' families of origin and past abuse. One foster daughter, Alice, whose problems were more serious (e.g., suicidal threats), was seeing an individual therapist weekly and had been doing so prior to her arrival in the Connors home. The parents cited their 20 years of fostering as evidence of their expertise in child rearing, while graciously agreeing that "of course, everyone can use some help sometimes." An atmosphere of pseudocooperation with this family therapy endeavor marked the interview, and it was difficult to discern just what the problems were that prompted the two referrals. A tone of protection was evident on the part of all family members, and the parents communicated a sense of hurt that they were being judged as incompetent foster parents, which was how they defined the referral for family therapy. An end-of-session assignment was given to clarify the aims of family therapy as far as the family was concerned, and an appointment was set for 2 weeks hence.

Mrs. Connors called on the day of the appointment and canceled, citing scheduling problems. She said she would call back when she knew their schedule, or the therapist could call her. In the meantime, the therapist began to receive calls from the two social workers urgently inquiring if therapy had ensued. Clearly, this family and the referral to family therapy were part of a complex family–larger system network that needed to be understood.

This example indicates the necessity for discerning and assessing the *meaningful system*, or that configuration of relationships and beliefs in which any given family's problems and issues make sense. To see the problem in the engagement process in this case as problems *in* the family leads one to notions of resistance, lack of cooperation, and so on. To formulate an assessment that examines the engagement process in the context of family–larger system relationships will enhance possibilities of effective engagement and relevant intervention in an appropriately wider network of relationships.

While assessment, interviewing, intervention, and evaluation are all interwoven aspects of a whole cloth, they are separated here for purposes of presenting a learnable model.

PURPOSES OF ASSESSMENT

The therapist seeks information regarding the place of larger systems in a particular family's life. Families who have engaged with larger helping systems for three generations with little hint of change in major patterns present a very different meaningful system for consideration than families whose involvement with larger helping systems is recent and temporary. Families who regard their history with larger systems as toxic or highly conflictual are obviously different from families who consider their relationships with helpers as benign or peaceful. Such differences may, however, upon further examination, be less marked at the level of whether change occurs. Miller (1983) in her work on families with alcohol problems suggests that seemingly angry relationships with larger systems and seemingly beneficent relationships with larger systems may well be adaptations with the same outcome, that of no new development or change.

The second purpose of assessment is to determine viable points of entry into the family sphere that do not replicate prior treatment attempts if these have proven pointless. A family with a long history with outside systems that have come to regard the family as hopeless or unworkable requires an engagement process that is free from such pessimistic predictions. One might find that all prior engagement was with the mother and an ill child, omitting the father, and that the father had become increasingly distant from *both* the family and the helping endeavor. With this information regarding the nature of prior family–larger system interaction, the therapist can plan a very different engagement that confirms the father's participation. Or a family who is involved with multiple agencies and who is being sent to family therapy, as in the Connors case, may require an engagement process that focuses first on their relationships with helpers rather than on individual members or their internal family relationships. Such a framing is often a refreshing surprise to families, since most families engaged with public-sector helpers are not asked about their experiences in this domain. Defining a family's problem at this level and focusing on their relationships with professional helpers often engages a family in a therapeutic endeavor designed to enhance their overall functioning such that multiple larger systems will deintensify their interest in the family.

This leads to the third purpose of assessment of family–larger system relationships, that of giving the therapist the possibility of creating and sustaining with the family a new and unanticipated relationship with a larger system. Once a therapist is able to assess the ongoing nature of the family–larger system relationship, he or she can avoid replicating this relationship once more. Such replication simply contributes to rigidity and reification both within the family and at the family–larger system interface. Thus in the Connors example, a therapist who did not attend to assessing the family–larger system configuration easily ran the risk of inadvertently allying with the social service system simply by agreeing to the referral and inquiring about problems. Since the family was experiencing social services as criticizing them via the referral for family therapy, a family therapist might be seen as joining these critical ranks.

Once a therapist begins to appreciate the past and present nature of family–larger system involvement, then he or she is in the position to plan and implement a *different* sort of relationship, one with unexpected elements capable of introducing new information. (See Chapter 6 for an elaboration of this concept of creating unanticipated relationships and the in-depth case illustration "A 40-Year Secret").

The fourth purpose of assessment is the maintenance of viable relationships with larger systems. Helpers in public-sector systems frequently experience disconfirmation from clients, other professionals, and their own systems. Such disconfirmation feeds cycles of symmetrical escalation regarding "who knows best" and contributes to cascading blame that ultimately harms clients. Family therapists have frequently been accused of discounting the valuable contributions of other professions or of being uncooperative. An atmosphere of mutual mistrust often marks the larger system network. When one carefully assesses the family–larger system macrosystem, one is far less likely to ascribe to notions of "good guys" and "bad guys" and will gain a sense of family–larger system interaction that is more circular and often stuck in ways that no one malevolently intends. The therapist is then able to appropriately confirm contributions of other professionals and initiate limited "partnerships" that draw upon distinct areas of knowledge.

The fifth purpose of assessment is to account for systemic constraints, or those elements in the family–larger system network that are presently unchangeable givens, regardless of intervention. When a therapist is not cognizant of such constraints, it is easy to contribute to the cynicism in the family with interventions or directions that are impossible to carry out, to begin viewing representatives of larger systems as villains when, in fact, they are most often doing the best job they can do in the given circumstances, or to blame oneself for ineffectiveness.

Often such constraints in the family–helper macrosystem are statutory. It behooves any therapist entering a community to become familiar with the range of laws that will effect therapeutic work. As laws and policies change, one needs knowledge of these changes and their potential effects in the therapeutic arena. For instance, the Connors foster family was sent for therapy at a time when state law was shifting and social workers, who previously were encouraged to develop permanent foster plans after 1 year of placement, were now being told to focus on reuniting families, resulting in a spate of referrals for family therapy without therapists being told of the underlying agenda (e.g., discovering "flaws" in the foster family that would make more palatable the plans to move a child back to his or her own home). Similarly, a therapist may be working with a natural family, self-referred, whose child is presently in foster care. If one lacks clear knowledge of current welfare policy, one may find that despite all attempts towards reunification desired by the family members, a legal and social policy process of "permanency planning" often precludes this outcome. Knowledge of such constraints can help the family therapist avoid work that will simply breed cynicism in families, and may lead the family therapist to important advocacy work at the social policy level.

A second area of constraint involves finances and the effects of governmental and insurance company decisions on the family–larger system network. In the 1980s such decisions have cut essential human services, often resulting in a situation where problems must be nearly unsolvable before intervention is available. For therapists working in the public sector, this has often meant working with an increasingly difficult population, whose problems are multiple and whose cynicism regarding the efficacy of help is appropriately high.

The issue of finances also provides a constraint regarding the popular third-party payment for therapeutic services. The therapeutic relationship immediately becomes one of three-party interaction, with a fair amount of mystification. Therapists may find that insurance companies are the salient and constraining larger systems regarding diagnostic labeling that contributes to reification (see Chapter 6 for a complete discussion of the labeling issue and case examples) or specifying a certain number of sessions.

Finances become an even more powerful and potentially damaging constraint, however, when a family is sent to therapy by a larger system that they consider to be a stressing agent upon them and the larger system is paying for the therapy and is hence expecting to "own" the outcome. The therapeutic alliance is easily compromised, as the family experiences the therapist as an ally of the larger system that is footing the bill. It is not unusual for the paying system to expect to set goals for treatment and to receive regular reports. A more general goal of any therapy, that of increased personal empowerment, may be readily sacrificed by a process that maintains the family in a dependent position as the real third party, existing between the payer and the payee.*

---

*In Canada, where some of this work is being written, everyone is entitled to universal health care, including therapeutic services. As of 1987 detailed reports or government goals for treatment outcome are not required. Thus, while a third-party payment system operates, it defines families as entitled to services by virtue of being participants in the society, rather than defining them as "one-down."

Too often there is no discussion of this financial issue, leaving it to exist as a silent, but potent, element in the family–larger system context, one that may constrain both therapeutic imagination and maneuverability.

Another area of constraint, frequently operative in the public-sector systems (e.g., welfare, probation, services for the handicapped, etc.), involves the rapid turnover of workers who interact with clients on the front line. It would not be unusual for a therapist working with a family involved with the welfare system to find that the family's social worker changes two or three times in 6 months. This seems to pertain all over North America. The effects of such shifts, whether due to burnout, frequent promotions, or geographic relocations, are to add elements of uncertainty to the family–larger system context, to mirror the very instability by which the families are frequently labeled, and to decrease motivation for problem solving, since the feedback circuit between the family and helpers, which could potentially provide affirmation, is constantly interrupted.

Knowledge of these various constraints in the family–larger system context, which become more visible with careful assessment, can assist the therapist to (1) demystify such constraints via frank discussion with any given family; (2) work where work is possible and not burn out attempting to deliver the undeliverable; (3) avoid unplanned alliances or splits with outside systems; and (4) make decisions about devoting a portion of one's professional time and energy to action at the social policy level.

The sixth purpose for assessment is leading the therapist to design and implement interventions in the family–larger system relationship, when it has been determined that this is the appropriate level for intervention. Understanding the salient patterns within the family, within the pertinent larger systems, and between family and larger systems, both historically and currently, opens the therapist's choices for intervention dramatically while avoiding intervention at the wrong level. Rather than curtailing interventions within the obvious boundaries of the family, which may be "more of the same wrong solution" (Watzlawick, Weakland, & Fisch, 1974), the therapist can intervene at the family–larger system interface, with particular combinations of family members and outsiders, or within the larger system per se, and potentiate effective change. Such expanded intervention options are especially pertinent when therapy has reached an impasse. (See Chapter 5 for a complete discussion of intervention design, implementation, and evaluation.)

The final purpose for assessment is to generate hypotheses pertaining to the place or function of particular families and for kinds of problems in and among larger systems.

Harrell (1980) notes that certain families come to function in enduring problematic patterns with larger systems and serve the function of reducing stress and conflict among the larger systems. Such "symptomatic" families or individuals may serve a homeostatic function within a particular larger system and between systems, reducing the necessity for change within the larger systems by consuming all the free energy and attention that might otherwise be focused on such internal needs. Approaching assessment at this level is especially efficacious when consulting directly to the larger systems (see Chapter 8).

Particular problems function to provide a *raison d'être* for certain larger systems. The identified problem and the larger system interact to define and support one another. Harkaway (1983) points to this interaction between the socially defined overweight and the bevy of larger systems that exist for weight reduction, in the face of clear evidence that such problems most frequently contribute to a diet–overeat cycle resulting in further weight gain. She cites how the programs of these systems fit with family interaction patterns vis-à-vis the "overweight symptom," making symptom resolution less and less likely. As one seeks to understand the function of whole categories of problems within families *and* larger systems, questions regarding the ways that problems and larger systems may perpetuate each other must be posed and ways out of this dilemma sought.

The purposes of assessing the family–larger system relationship can thus be enumerated as follows:

1. To provide information regarding the place of larger systems in a family's life, leading to hypotheses regarding the *meaningful system* for intervention.
2. To determine viable points of entry in the family sphere.
3. To create new and unanticipated relationships between a family and larger system, thereby making a change process more viable.
4. To maintain viable relationships with larger systems.
5. To determine constraints in the family–larger system context.
6. To contribute to intervention design and implementation at the appropriate level.
7. To provide information regarding the place of particular families and problems in and among larger systems, in order to facilitate effective program development.

ELEMENTS OF ASSESSMENT

The family therapist wanting to assess family–larger system relationships should attend to several elements, including (1) determining which systems are involved, (2) problem definitions among the various salient systems, (3) dyadic and triadic arrangements between the family and larger systems, (4) boundaries between the family and larger systems, (5) myths and beliefs, (6) past and current solution behavior, (7) binds, (8) transitions in the macrosystems, and (9) predictions.

Contributions to the assessment process come from specific information gathered from the family, from the referral source and other larger systems interacting with the family, from conducting a family–larger system interview (see Chapter 4), and from one's general fund of knowledge regarding the behavior of specific larger systems, as required by law and policy and as idiosyncratically translated by particular workers. The assessment process will unfold and change throughout therapy, as more information becomes available and the interaction of family and larger systems responds to the therapeutic context. A family therapist will find it efficacious to devote a portion of a first interview to an inquiry regarding the family's relationship to larger systems. Such an inquiry will likely yield hypotheses and a direction for entry and subsequent therapeutic action that would not otherwise be available.

Determining Which Larger Systems Are Involved

Assessment begins with determining which larger systems are involved with the family. Gathering such information immediately begins to provide the skeletal features of a family–larger system map. One is interested first in which and how may agencies regularly interact with the family. A given agency may have several subsystems that are involved with various parts of a family or may present diverse agendas to the family and to each other. One is interested, too, in how long the family has been involved with these or other outside systems.

Returning to the Connors family, one can see how the question of past and current involvement with larger systems expands one's understanding of the meaningful system.

CASE EXAMPLE (CONTINUED)

In the first session with the Connors family, the family therapist asked questions about outside systems and determined that the parents had regularly interacted with government social services for the entire length of their marriage, as they had begun to take in foster children as a young couple 20 years earlier. Since they had fostered 15 children and since workers often were changed for a given child, they estimated that they had related with 35 social workers for the children, as well as about a half dozen eligibility workers who were supposed to enter the family sphere every 6 months to reestablish their eligibility as a foster family and determine their financial remuneration. Thirteen-year-old Alice also had an individual therapist to whom she was referred 2 years ago by her social worker. She saw this therapist weekly.

Inquiries about the extended family's interactions with larger systems revealed that both Mr. and Mrs. Connors's families were overseas and neither could recall any regular interactions with larger systems, other than church, which they both stipulated bore no similarity to their situation.

The nuclear family genogram is one small part of the complex Connors family–larger system genogram, shown in Figure 3-1. Questions arise about the nature of family–larger system interaction, about the effects on family life and identity of such regular involvement with outside systems, about methods that the family has designed in order to exist in their network, about how the family is regarded by the outside systems, and about what it means that this family's extended family did not interact with public-sector systems. The time required to gather the above material is about 15 minutes. The hypotheses that begin to be generated will help shape the course of therapy and will help defuse traps and struggles that frequently emerge when a family is engaged with outside systems as this family is.

The initial question regarding what larger systems are involved begins to branch off in several directions. One is interested in current and past involvement. A family may, for instance, have no other current involvement with outsiders and be self-referred for family therapy. When one inquires about past involvement with larger systems, however, one may discover that the family has had three failed attempts at family treatment or that the father had individual therapy for 5 years, which the mother resented and that the current family therapy is his attempt to get her into treatment, or conversely that the family had a very good experience earlier in their history with therapy and that they are approaching the present endeavor with hope. All of these factors form a contextual backdrop for any new engagement with a larger system and are information that can be gathered in a very brief time.

In gathering information about the family's involvement with outsiders, one is interested in both temporal and numerical dimensions. Has the family, or a member, been involved with one outsider, such as a physician or therapist, for 10 or 20 years? If so, this outsider may have become like a family member (Selvini-Palazzoli et al., 1980b). Or has the family rapidly enlisted a dozen outsiders within the last 6 months, when previously they had interacted with none? The temporal issue can also be examined within a family life-cycle perspective in order to determine if the family is one that interacts with larger systems at particular life-cycle transitions, such as children leaving home, or whether every aspect of the family's life cycle involves outside systems, as in the Connors case.

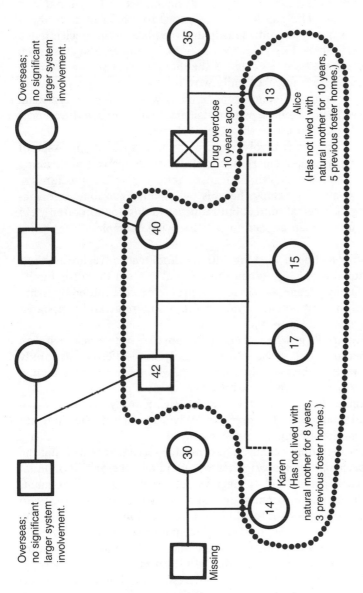

Overseas;
no significant
larger system
involvement.

Overseas;
no significant
larger system
involvement.

35

13

Drug overdose
10 years ago.

Alice
(Has not lived with
natural mother for 10 years,
5 previous foster homes.)

40

42

15

17

30

Karen
(Has not lived with
natural mother for 8 years,
3 previous foster homes.)

14

Missing

Past Systems: Government social services — 30 to 40 workers over 20 years
Present Systems: Government social services — 3 workers
Mental health — 1 therapist for Alice for 2 years
Family therapy clinic — 2 therapists

Figure 3-1. The Connors family genogram and larger system involvement.

53

Questions regarding involvement with larger systems may also yield a picture in which the family has had absolutely no involvement with outside systems other than routine involvement with educational and health care systems. This can lead the therapist to a brief inquiry about the current decision to seek outside help and the place of this decision in a context formerly shaped by rules that may have mitigated against such involvement. Soon it becomes clear to the therapist that such a family is different in many ways from a family with a 20-year history with larger systems, that both are different from families with a multigenerational legacy of negative involvement with outsiders, and that such differences can be put to beneficial use in the present therapy.

In the area of current involvement with larger systems, the issue of the present referral source emerges, coupled with the perceived meaning of the referral and the overall pattern of referring within the family–larger system context. A family therapist will likely have some information regarding the referral source, but inquiries in this domain often yield surprising results, as can be seen in the following examples:

1. A family had been working with a school teacher regarding their son's educational problems. When the teacher referred them for family therapy, the family felt she was saying the problems were caused by them. They canceled the first two appointments and only reluctantly appeared for the third when this issue was discovered.

2. A 15-year-old girl had been in therapy for over a year with an individual therapist. When she and her family were referred for family therapy, she believed the individual therapist, whom she regarded highly, was angry with her and was punishing her for slow progress.

3. A woman had confided in her physician for years, discussing severe marital conflicts and depression. When he referred her and her husband for marital therapy, she felt betrayed.

4. Inquiry regarding a family's referrals for services revealed that the family had been *simultaneously* referred for family therapy, individual therapy for each parent and teenage child, psychological assessment, alcohol treatment, and a parent support group by the same worker, who was praised by her supervisor for doing a thorough job. Not surprisingly, the family turned up for family therapy feeling resentful and frazzled.

5. Two larger systems, mental health and child welfare, were simultaneously involved with a family. Mental health provided play therapy, while child welfare had a supervisory interest in the family. The child-welfare worker was not pleased with the work of the mental health agency, and vice versa. Subtle battles over "who knows best" were rife. Without informing the mental health agency, the family was referred by the child-welfare worker for family therapy, opening the potential triangle before family treatment even ensued.

CASE EXAMPLE (CONTINUED)

The referral pattern with the Connors family was complicated. Each of the foster daughters' social workers had opted for a referral to family therapy. Neither had been terribly clear with the family regarding the reasons for referral, and neither had informed the family's eligibility worker or Alice's therapist of the decision. The family had become used to Alice going to therapy and believed this was appropriate, since she had severe individual problems. The family regarded the family therapy referral as criticism of their family and an indication that somebody believed they had severe problems as a family, which they denied. The referral sources' purposes remained veiled until a family–larger system interview was conducted at the second session.

In addition to the intentions of the referral source and the meanings ascribed to the referral by the family and other involved systems, one is also interested in the overall pattern of referral. Were referrals for several different services made simultaneously? Has the particular family been passed from one agency to another over a period of months or years? Does the referral source refer and back off or refer and hold on? What sort of reporting is expected, and what does the family understand about this process? Is referral part of an ongoing struggle between two or more outside systems?

The following questions are useful in determining which larger systems are involved; the second column represents answers from the first interview with the Connors family.

What larger systems are involved with the family?	The Connors family is involved with social services and community mental health.
How many agencies regularly interact with the family?	Two major agencies, but three ongoing workers; social services involvement includes two subsystems, child welfare and eligibility.
For how long and with what frequency?	For 20 years at least monthly, often more.
What is the family's history with larger systems?	Social services has had lots of involvement with the nuclear family. The extended family has had no larger system involvement.
What is the current involvement with larger systems?	Involved with social services, community mental health, and a family therapist.

How have the referral sources inter-acted with the family (intentions, meanings)?	The family sees the referral sources as critical. Other referral information is missing; find out about referrals interaction.

Definitions of the Problem

When a family is engaged with larger systems, determining how the family and outsiders define the problem or problems is crucial both to understanding the family–larger system relationship and to the subsequent course of therapeutic work. A variety of possible configurations appear. The family and outsiders may be in total agreement, or they may agree about the problem but disagree on the ways to deal with it. Or there may be lots of conflict about the very nature of the problem. A symmetrically escalating battle may ensue regarding either the problem definition, the suggestion of family therapy, or both. Various alliances and splits may emerge, as certain family members and certain helpers join in particular definitions. Such patterns may be metaphorical, representing the overall pattern of relationship between the family and larger systems. In the case under discussion, the Connorses and social services held distinctly different definitions of the problem.

CASE EXAMPLE (CONTINUED)

When the Connors family was referred for family therapy, all of the family firmly expressed the belief that Alice was the problem, that her behavior was explainable by her traumatic history prior to her current foster placement, and that individual therapy for Alice, while not yet yielding results, was the preferred approach. Conversely, the two social workers believed that, while both Karen and Alice had problems stemming from their pasts, these problems were escalating and that therefore their current context required treatment. Gradually information emerged that the eligibility worker did not favor the referral for family therapy and agreed with the parents that individual therapy for Alice should continue. Alice's therapist agreed. Thus, even before family therapy began, a triangle existed in the family–larger system network over definition of the problem (see Figure 3-2). A family therapist might easily be drawn into the fray.

Definitions of the problem are shaped by larger system mandates. The same behavior, for instance stealing by an adolescent, may be defined as bad or "criminal" behavior by a probation department, as "sinful" behavior by a church, and as "psychologically troubled" behav-

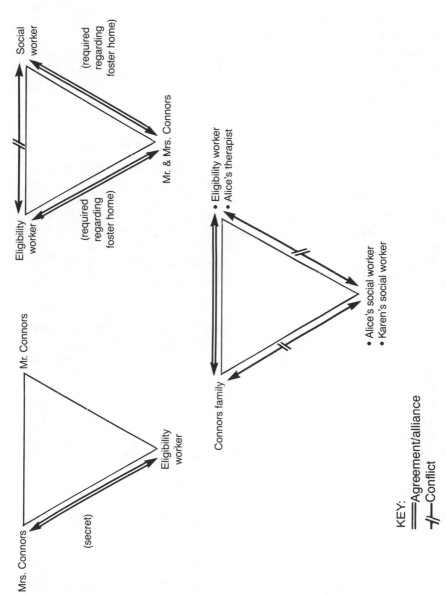

KEY:
═══ Agreement/alliance
─//─ Conflict

Figure 3-2. Connors family and larger system triangulation regarding definition of the problem and perceived solution.

ior by a school system involved with parent education. One may see markedly different definitions of the same case, or one may see cases routed to specific systems due to class and racial prejudice. In many communities, truant behavior by a wealthy boy will result in psychological referrals, while the same behavior in a poor youngster will result in delinquency referrals. All such definitions shape and direct subsequent beliefs and intervention attempts. As specific mandates of the larger systems shift, so too will definitions of the problem, as can be seen in the Connors case.

CASE EXAMPLE (CONTINUED)

When the Connors were referred for family therapy, the specific mandate of social services was undergoing a profound shift that instructed workers to focus on family dynamics and interaction in all aspects of their work. The same worker who had previously referred Alice for individual therapy was now seeking to understand Alice's problems from a family perspective. This ran counter to what the Connorses had previously been led to believe about Alice from the same larger system. The Connorses had no information regarding this mandate shift. They felt both mystified and blamed.

As one seeks definitions of the problem, often the preferred locus of blame is illuminated. Helpers may be nonblameful; may blame the entire family for some shortcoming; may place blame on one family member, the marriage, or the parenting style; or may blame other helpers. The family, in turn, may blame their own unit or specific members or may place subtle or blatant blame on the outside systems. Such blame placing may operate to unite or split segments of the macrosystem, as when a school blames a child and the family responds by either joining in blaming the child or uniting with the child to blame the school.

CASE EXAMPLE (CONTINUED)

The Connors family outwardly placed blame for their predicament on Alice's background, her natural mother, and previous foster placements. More subtly, however, they blamed the two social workers and Alice's individual therapist for not solving Alice's problems. They saw themselves as blame-free, citing their years as foster parents as evidence. The two social workers, however, felt something was amiss in the foster home and at the family–larger system interview blamed Alice's problems on unresolved marital issues of Mr. and Mrs. Connors, stating that this was contributing to an atmosphere of instability. As this information, previously unknown to the therapist, emerged, Mr. and Mrs. Connors countered with information regarding the reappearance of Alice's natural mother and her harmful effect on Alice. Thus the family and larger systems were divided regarding locus of blame, and each one's explanations engendered defensiveness and further blaming in the other, in an escalating symmetrical pattern.

Discussions of the definition of the problem will yield a tone of calm, or urgency, or boredom, or crisis that may differ among the various participants. Outside systems may be much more upset or worried by a situation than the family appears to be. The family may present as if you looked them up in the telephone directory and invited them in, or express confusion, or indicate that they are not having great difficulties, while outside systems appear to be in a panic. If a therapist gets caught in the outside system's attitude of worry, panic, or heightened concern, he or she may quickly become allied with the outside systems and part of an escalating complementary pattern in which the family appears more and more sedate, while the larger systems become more frantic.

A family may be having little or no trouble with a youngster whom a school teacher is finding impossible. The therapist should discover whether the meaningful system for intervention is (1) the child, who may, for instance, be exhibiting a neurological problem; (2) the family, whose child for some reason is behaving in unusual ways in the outside world; (3) the parent, school, and child configuration; (4) the particular classroom or school system; or (5) some combination of these. The problem may or may not be best resolved in the family's context or may require the presence of outside systems for resolutions.

CASE EXAMPLE (CONTINUED)

The Connors family appeared fairly calm and understated regarding the problems with Alice, who had engaged in several self-destructive episodes. They analyzed this behavior in a context that included their long experience as foster parents for emotionally disturbed children and saw Alice as no worse than many. They dismissed Karen's problems as quite routine. Meanwhile, Alice's social worker was extremely alarmed over what she saw as suicidal behavior on Alice's part. Her concern was exacerbated by the family's calm approach. Karen's social worker was very upset over Karen's poor hygiene and referred Karen for a psychiatric evaluation prior to the family therapy referral. The larger system was clearly more upset than the family and became more and more upset as the family appeared untroubled by the circumstances.

Preferred definitions of the problem, accompanied by referrals for family therapy, may hold hidden agendas that larger systems have for a family or that a family may have vis-à-vis a larger system. A larger system may send a family for treatment regarding a child, with the hidden agenda of discovering information about the family or the marital pair. A family may accept referral after referral, with the hidden agenda of proving a problem is unsolvable and extruding a member. Hidden agendas often become visible during thorough investigations of various definitions of the problem, as occurred in the Connors case.

CASE EXAMPLE (CONTINUED)

During the second interview, which included representatives of the larger systems, Alice's social worker stated several times, "I just don't know the Connors family very well. I don't seem to be able to get to know them as I have my other families." When this comment was investigated, her hidden agenda, that of sending the family for therapy in order to receive ongoing reports, emerged. Karen's social worker, in answer to questions about her concerns that went beyond Karen, revealed that she had heard from the eligibility worker that Mr. and Mrs. Connors were having marital problems and that Mr. Connors had had an affair. Her hidden agenda, which the Connorses clearly sensed but had not brought up, was for the Connorses to receive unasked-for marital therapy.

The following questions are useful in defining the problem; the second column represents answers from a second interview, with the Connors family and representatives of the larger systems.

How do the family and larger systems define the problem and appropriate approaches?	The family, the eligibility worker, and the individual therapist believe the problem is Alice and the appropriate approach is individual therapy; Alice's and Karen's social workers believe the family has a problem and the appropriate approach is family therapy.
Do larger system mandates shape the definition of the problem?	The social services mandate to focus on families contributes to their view that the Connorses need help.
Are there any areas of agreement?	No.
What are the various configurations of disagreement?	The family, eligibility worker, and individual therapist are aligned against the two social workers.

What is the preferred locus of blame?	The family blames social services, the individual therapist, Alice, and Alice's mother; the social workers blame the family.
Whose problem is it, anyway?	Social services is *much* more upset than the family appears to be.
Are there hidden agendas?	The social workers' hidden agenda is to secure marital therapy for Mr. and Mrs. Connors and to receive reports on information that they are unable to gather.

Dyads and Triads

While certain dyadic and triadic arrangements may emerge only in the parties' definitions of the problem, as described above, many families and larger systems exist in enduring dyads and triads, forming rigid patterns that may be metaphors for patterns within the family and the larger system. Assessment of these patterns is essential for subsequent interviewing, intervention design, and implementation (as will be demonstrated in Chapters 4, 5, and 6).

Symmetry and Complementarity

The theoretical constructs of *complementarity* and *symmetry* (Bateson, 1972, 1979; Lederer & Jackson, 1968; Watzlawick, Beavin, & Jackson, 1967) generally applied to simple dyads, most often husband and wife, are extremely useful for examining the patterns that develop either between individual family members and larger system representatives or between whole families as a unit and larger systems. In his early anthropological work in New Guinea, Bateson (1979), noted

> that various relations among groups and among various types of kin were characterized by interchanges of behavior such that the more A exhibited a given behavior, the more B was likely to exhibit the same behavior. These I called *symmetrical* interchanges. Conversely, there were also stylized interchanges in which B's behavior was different from, but *complementary* to that of A. In either case the relations were more potentially subject to progressive escalation. (p. 105)

Thus, in the family–larger system assessment, one may examine relationships for complementarity, symmetry, escalating complementarity, and escalating symmetry.

Such patterns at the family–larger system level frequently reflect patterns within the family, within the larger system, or between larger systems. For instance, if the couple in a family exist in an enduring symmetrically escalating relationship, it is not unusual to see such symmetrical escalation reflected between the couple and the helpers. Such symmetry may show itself in struggles over the nature of help offered, whether and when to make appointments, and so on. Such symmetry may then extend throughout the larger system, as when a couple fighting with each other and symmetrically exchanging angry responses, begin to fight with their helper, who in turn argues with his supervisor, who then invites in and argues with a consultant. Or one may see a symmetrically escalating couple line up a bevy of helpers on each side, who do battle with each other in a pattern that is isomorphic with the couple's pattern. In one case a wife had a welfare worker, a school counselor, and a shelter worker on her side, while the husband had a probation officer, an individual therapist, and the police on his side, and the various workers symmetrically struggled just as the couple did.

One may also see such isomorphism with escalating complementarity. A family may define one member, for instance a single parent, as helpless. If outside systems enter, also define her as helpless, and begin to add more and more helpers, the escalating complementarity within the family will be mirrored between the family and larger systems. Another example is the situation where a couple's escalating complementarity shows itself in one parent, often the mother in our culture, becoming very worried or concerned about a child's behavior. Her worry is met with a complementary response by her husband, who shows no worry and counsels calm and optimism. The more he appears unruffled, the more frantic she appears, and each one's response provokes a further escalation. Any larger system entering runs the risk of joining this escalating complementarity: If a helper expresses a lot of worry, it is likely that the father will withdraw more, and if the helper is nonchalant, it is likely that the mother will find cause to worry more or may seek another helper, thus generating a multiple-helper situation where the escalating complementarity of worry and calm will prevail. (The "Family born with larger systems" case, described in Chapter 2, exemplifies this pattern.)

Symmetrical and complementary struggles may also exist within a given larger system or between larger systems and be reflected in the family–larger system network. Thus, if two larger systems such as mental health and child welfare routinely have symmetrical exchanges regarding who knows best, decision making, or types of treatment, such symmetry may be reflected in their relationships with a particular family. This pattern may be seen in the larger system interacting with the Connorses.

CASE EXAMPLE (CONTINUED)

The larger system, social services, with whom the Connors were involved had historically existed with symmetrical struggles between the child-welfare component and the foster care eligibility component. Further, at the time of referral of the Connors family, a symmetrically escalating battle between mental health and social services had been going on for about 2 years. While this battle was being fought at state and regional administrative levels over issues of funding, mandates, and confidentiality, individual workers at the local level were keenly aware of the fights and of the ongoing symmetrical attacks between the systems. Thus, the macrosystem within which the Connors family existed and was being treated was permeated with patterns of symmetrical escalation across a variety of content areas. The symmetrical struggle regarding family therapy, both between the family and the social workers and among the various helpers, was a familiar struggle to all concerned. Without change in the nature of this struggle, no new information would enter the ecosystem at a pattern level. Further, if the family therapist began to similarly struggle with either the family or the larger systems regarding the efficacy of family therapy, the symmetrical pattern would continue.

The issue of complementarity and symmetry between families and larger systems must also be set in the context of the socially accepted definition of the helping endeavor in our culture. Professional help is generally predefined as a complementary relationship between helper and helpee.* If either party does not accept this definition, then a symmetrical struggle may quickly ensue regarding the definition of the relationship.

CASE EXAMPLE (CONTINUED)

In the case of the Connorses, social services was defining the family as clients in a complementary relationship of helpers and clients, in which experts offer guidance to clients, who accept such guidance. Mr. and Mrs. Connors, however, defined the relationship as symmetrical, seeing themselves as partners with social services in the provision of foster care. Further, they viewed their 20-year history as foster parents as imparting expertise to them, both about foster children *and* about social workers. As each side pushed their definition of the relationship, escalating symmetry prevailed.

*An exception to this complementary definition is feminist therapy, which explicitly defines the therapeutic relationship as symmetrical. Since feminist therapy exists, however, within a broader cultural context that defines therapy as complementary, this explicit symmetrical definition may engender mystification.

The symmetrical and/or complementary nature of the relationship between families and larger systems may be embedded in particular themes. In the Connors's relationship with larger systems, escalating symmetry pertained regarding the theme of "help," but a pattern of escalating complementarity prevailed regarding the theme of "worry" as the social workers showed more and more worry and the family displayed more and more dispassion.

During the second session, when the helpers were present, both patterns were evident. The family and the helpers symmetrically struggled over whether or not the family needed help and the nature of such help. As the helpers listed their various concerns about the family, including marital conflict and sibling problems, the family responded with more and more assurance that such problems were solved and cited that, after the first family therapy session, all of the children became enormously more cooperative, proving that further help was not needed. With each presentation by the family that all was well, the social workers voiced further concerns, which were met with more evidence from the family that all was well. The unfortunate nature of this escalation seemed to require that the family not ask for help even if they felt help was needed, as for the marital problems.

Complementarity and symmetry can be examined in the family–larger system network from a number of vantage points (specifics for the Connors family are in the second column).

Are there prevailing and escalating patterns of complementarity and/or symmetry between the family and larger systems?	Yes.
Are such patterns isomorphic with patterns within the family, within the larger system, and/or between larger systems?	Symmetrical escalation between the Connors family and larger systems is isomorphic with escalating symmetry between subsystems in social services and between social services and mental health.
Are the patterns in synchrony with or in conflict with implicit definitions shaping client–helper relationships?	In conflict.
What themes underpin the patterns?	Themes of help and worry.

Triads

The triadic combinations among families and larger systems are legion, involving alliances and splits between whole families and larger systems, among individual family members and specific representatives of larger systems, and among various larger systems. As one moves from dyadic analysis to triadic analysis, the organizational level emerges and with it issues of power, secrecy, deleterious effects on family and larger system functioning, and the ever-increasing likelihood of being drawn inadvertently into preexisting triangles.

Just as in dyadic arrangements, triadic patterns may mirror family process. A couple that is familiar with three-party interaction will easily form triangles with outside systems. Helpers who do not stop to assess the wider picture may easily form alliances and splits with family members, perpetuating internal family triangles. A family in which the mother and a handicapped child are allied and the father is more distant from both wife and child may find that the larger helping systems perpetuate and exacerbate this pattern by interacting with and supporting the mother at the expense of the parental dyad. This may begin at the child's birth and is easily promoted by the social view that the child's problems are the province of the mother. Appointments are set when the father cannot come, the mother's expertise about the child's problems grows, the father is omitted and omits himself more and more, and the mother grows closer to professional helpers, increasingly turning to them rather than to her husband (Imber-Black, 1986d; Imber Coppersmith, 1982b).

A family in which parents are split and form triangles with children as allies may form similar triangles with multiple helpers as allies, such that each parent has an alliance with one or more helpers. The Moore family, described in "A family born with larger systems," in which a dietician was allied with the mother and maternal grandmother, a physician was allied with the father and paternal grandmother, and the child was unable to side with one without risking disloyalty to the other, is a prime example of this process.

Families may also become parts of larger system triangles. An examination of families who were chronically and unsuccessfully involved with public-sector systems over several generations revealed that such families were part of enduring triads, characterized either by conflictual relationships among the several systems "helping" the family or by conflictual triads formed by the family members and helpers (Harrell, 1980).

The three triadic patterns—detour, cross-generational coalition, and triangulation—defined by Minuchin (1974) as pertaining to families are useful, with modification and expansion, in analysis of family–larger system triads.

The *detour* process may operate in two ways. First, one may see otherwise conflictual larger systems, or subsystems within a given larger system, unite either in anger or overprotection regarding a particular family. Here it is important to know the history and the ongoing nature of relationships among larger systems in a given community. It is not unusual to discover a persistent enmity and mistrust between a child-welfare system and mental health system, between a public school and a private school dealing with handicapped children, or between a day hospital component and an outpatient component of a large community mental health system. In the midst of usual negative interactions, when participants in these systems suddenly submerge their differences regarding a particular family in ways that either scapegoat or offer pity, a detour is likely in progress.

In the second detour process, family members may be able to ignore internal conflicts by focusing their concerns on outside systems. Such detouring may be the continuation of a familiar internal pattern, as when a conflicted couple has united for many years to attack a child who, in turn, has given them frequent cause for anger. When this child moves out, the husband and wife begin to engage with outside systems in a process that begins with complaints about the other spouse and moves rapidly to both spouses uniting to attack the various helpers as incompetent. The larger systems inadvertently step into the void left by the absent child, thereby maintaining the familiar detour pattern.

One may also see such detouring in response to recent, unmanageable conflict or pain in a family. The rapid enlistment of several outsiders, none of whom are satisfactory and who draw the collective ire of the family, is often an indicator of such detouring.

What Minuchin refers to as cross-generational coalition is here renamed as *cross-system coalition*, a pattern where individual family members form alliances with members of outside systems. Such alliances may either exclude or be patently against other family members and other helpers and hence may preclude problem resolution or exacerbate problems. A common cross-system alliance occurs when one spouse and a helper focus on the shortcomings of the other spouse. Such an arrangement often involves secrecy. The complaining spouse may readily come to feel more understood and supported by the helper than by the other spouse, contributing to a deterioration in the marriage.

CASE EXAMPLE (CONTINUED)

In the Connors family, Mrs. Connors interacted frequently and intensely with the eligibility worker. While the eligibility worker's defined role was to contact the family every 6 months, in fact she and Mrs. Connors spoke by telephone weekly regarding problems in the family and in the marriage. When Mr. Connors had an extramarital affair, Mrs. Connors turned to the eligibility worker to discuss it. These conversations were secret from Mr. Connors, thus placing more distance between the couple and precluding effective resolution of the issue. Mrs. Connors assumed the information regarding the affair was also secret from the other social workers, but the eligibility worker felt she had to impart this information to them, forming other secret alliances. Since the social workers were not at liberty to raise this issue with the Connorses, all communication between them became more mystified, resulting in the referral for family therapy, a veiled attempt to drive the marital issues into the open. Seen from this perspective, the eligibility worker's negative stance towards family therapy begins to make more sense, as she was in a position that required her to protect both Mrs. Connors and herself.

Cross-system alliances are frequently seen between adolescents and youth workers who form alliances against "old-fashioned" parents. An example of this pattern is a situation where an increasingly delinquent adolescent girl was intensely allied with both a youth worker and a school counselor. Whenever the girl's parents set rules for her, she complained bitterly to her youth worker and counselor, who would join and telephone the parents, reprimanding them for not treating the girl as a young adult. By the time the family came for family therapy, the parents felt hopeless, powerless, and disgusted with the larger systems. The girl's escalating delinquency functioned to maintain the alliances with the youth worker and the counselor. Similarly, an alliance between a child and a Big Brother may operate to disempower a single parent. Possible solutions to problems within the family are short-circuited by the potential for disloyalty to the cross-system alliance.

In *triangulation* a family may exist in two incompatible alliances with larger systems, or components of a larger system, that are in conflict with one another. The larger systems may fight over the definition of the family's problem and the preferred solution. Here family therapists have often entered the fray by struggling with helpers who are urging other treatments. If a family is required to be involved with the two or more larger systems that are in conflict (e.g., welfare and public school or two physicians), it may find itself in a fierce loyalty bind, not unlike the triangulation of two parents and a child. Like triangulation in families, this pattern between families and larger systems supports a communication process marked by mystification, disqualification of self and others, and a reduced capacity to discern locus of responsibility (Imber Coppersmith, 1985b).

CASE EXAMPLE (CONTINUED)

The Connorses were required to maintain alliances with two parts of the social services system, foster care eligibility and child welfare. The specific mandates of these two components, that is, finding and maintaining foster families, which are a scarce commodity, and protecting children, while sometimes compatible, are often not, since the primary concerns differ. The eligibility worker was more inclined to be understanding towards the family in an effort to preserve a 20-year relationship, while the social workers were more willing to see flaws in the family if they believed these were affecting the children. The conflicts between the two components were subtle but actual, and cut across many cases as a pervasive theme. The Connors's united front and air of pseudocooperation with the family therapy endeavor began to make sense as a response to their position in this pattern of triangulation. Comments from the parents like "Everybody can use some help some time," which placed them neither for nor against family therapy, are typical remarks that emerge in such patterns.

Larger systems per se may also form the various triadic patterns discussed above, irrespective of clients or families. This framework may be used for analysis by consultants to the larger systems. (See Chapter 8 for a complete discussion of such consultation.)

When examining triads formed between family members and helpers, it is important to factor in the issue of power. Many times, triads in the macrosystem are *not* equilateral, in the sense of simply being equal interacting parts of a system. Rather, the larger system may have power to influence and effect outcomes that a family lacks. Such power may be statutory, such as welfare laws, or may reside in bureaucratic trappings that a family alone finds impossible to overcome. Interventions here involve the thoughtful and deliberate formation of alliance for the purposes of coaching and advocacy (discussed in Chapter 6).

An analysis of triads in the macrosystem is especially crucial as the family therapist enters, in order to avoid joining preexisting patterns of alliances and splits and thereby contributing to rigidity in the macrosystem.

Triadic patterns form an important level of analysis of the family–larger system relationship. Assessment may include the following questions (specifics for the Connors family are in the second column).

What triads are formed by the family and larger systems?	See Figure 3-2.
What are the specific patterns?	Two patterns are operating in the Connors case, cross-system alliance and triangulation.
How is the family–larger system functioning affected by the triadic arrangements?	Mystification and disqualification of oneself as the locus of responsible action have increased. Spouse subsystem problem solving has decreased.

	Struggles within the larger system have increased.
What is the potential for the family therapist to inadvertently join triads?	The therapist is pulled to ally both by the family and the larger system.

Boundaries

The boundaries between a family and larger systems may be too diffuse, handicapping the family's coping resources, or too rigid, preventing the utilization of necessary assistance or the entry of new information. Boundaries between families and larger systems do not necessarily reflect the family's internal boundaries; families with diffuse interpersonal boundaries may draw a rigid boundary to the outside world, as for instance in families with incest, while families with rigid interpersonal boundaries may create intense relationships involving diffuse boundaries with outside helpers.

Boundaries are interactional phenomena, requiring participation of both family and larger system for their establishment and maintenance. However, individual families do influence the establishment of boundaries vis-à-vis the outside world in general and larger helping systems in particular. Such boundaries are often indicated metaphorically by physical aspects of the household (Miller, 1983). A family, seen many years ago by an outreach project, that had many agencies attempting to gain access had a sign on the lawn, "Do not ring doorbell or the dog will bite you," and an in–out board for family members on the front porch. Certainly the family was making a statement to the outside world about the nature of family–larger system boundaries. Paradoxically, families with such rigid boundaries to the outside world may find themselves recipients of the very intrusion that they abjure.

Likewise, particular larger systems function in ways that are more intrusive than others, generally because of their mandate, beliefs, and past experiences. It is not unusual to find a child-welfare system entering a widening circle of concerns in a family, under the mandate of child protection, which frequently allows investigation of all aspects of a family's life. Critical past experiences where children were endangered often fuel the worker's need to know more and more about a family. Many larger systems easily overstep the bounds of their mandates, as when school teachers begin to investigate a marriage or a child's social worker becomes a parent's confidante, as in the case under discussion. Families frequently do not know what boundaries they may allowably draw vis-à-vis public-sector systems and may share information when that is not in their best interest. (See Chapter 6 for a discussion of coaching as an intervention.)

When family–larger system boundaries are too diffuse, larger systems may define a family's problems for the family, become entangled in aspects of the family's life that are not their purview, gain access to areas of the family's life that would ordinarily be more private, and alternate between overprotecting family members and becoming exasperated with them.

Rigid boundaries may be characterized by a family's stereotyped denial of entry to other systems and their isolation from extrafamilial sources of information. Rigid boundaries may also arise when families cannot gain access to needed services because of class or racial issues. Sometimes such rigid boundaries are subtle and implicit, seen only when statistical analysis reveals, for instance, that Native American families are not served or are underserved at a local community mental health system, while showing up in large numbers on probation roles. Boundaries between various larger systems also affect the family–larger system relationship. Some larger systems have very diffuse boundaries, characterized by gossip or the sharing of information about families or other workers that is not relevant to the issue at hand. They may expect reports about the family to reveal information that the family would not tell them directly. Some larger systems have more rigid boundaries to other larger systems and may refuse to share information even when permission has been given to do so. The various boundary negotiations among larger systems in a community affect the families with which these systems are involved.

The sheer number of larger systems involved with or attempting to be involved with a family is not a clear indication of boundaries. A family may be involved with only one larger system, for instance health care delivery, yet a single representative of that system may have become like a member of the family. Conversely, a family may have six larger systems attempting, but failing, to gain access.

Particular problems arise when a larger system has one view of boundaries and the family has a different view. This may occur either when a larger system wants more diffuse boundaries, desiring access to information about the family, while the family wants more rigid boundaries, restricting such access, or when the family wants more access to the larger system than it is willing to give. In the first situation, the larger system may escalate its attempts to gain entry and be met with more refusal from the family. In any case it is likely that the system desiring more diffuse boundaries will go in search of allies to support its efforts.

In examining family–larger system boundaries, it is important to draw a distinction between families that have temporary relationships with larger systems and families that, because of long-lasting conditions, including, illness, handicaps, or poverty, must exist in enduring relationships with larger systems. The latter families must alter their boundaries to the outside world in ways that are more permanent, accommodating multiple larger systems in their sphere while simultaneously accommodating to a chronic condition.

Families, especially those that had been private, isolated, or otherwise disengaged from large, formal systems, may have a difficult time as larger systems initially enter. If such families begin the relationship by distancing from the larger system, this action may easily be misunderstood as a lack of interest in their ill member, or hostility, rather than an initial difficulty in altering boundaries. If the larger system distances in turn, as often happens, then a macrosystem marked by rigid, impermeable boundaries may develop.

Families with required enduring relationships with larger systems will often "appoint" one member to deal with the helpers. This person may be seen as negotiating the family's boundary with larger systems. Frequently this person, often the mother, gets designated as "overinvolved," rather than assessed as occupying a necessary position.

CASE EXAMPLE (CONTINUED)

Unlike most families, the Connorses had an ongoing boundary between their family and social services. Consequently, many aspects of family life that would normally be private were scrutinized by the larger system. The family's response to this was that Mrs. Conners was the primary boundary negotiator for the family. She handled all of the interactions with social services. The boundary between the family and the eligibility component of social services was quite diffuse, as the eligibility worker was given and sought information well beyond her mandate. In turn, this information was secretly shared with the child-welfare component, whose boundary with the family was generally more rigid and circumscribed to foster child issues. As the child-welfare workers sought a more diffuse boundary with the family, the family responded by giving them less and less information. Several times during the family–larger system interview, one of the child-welfare workers commented, "I just don't feel I *know* the Connors family, and I'm not comfortable with that." At this juncture, the child-welfare workers went in search of an ally in the family therapist. At the family–larger system interview, the child-welfare workers indicated that they expected regular reports from the family therapist. This expectation can be seen as their attempt to negotiate indirectly a more diffuse boundary.

Boundaries between families and larger systems monitor the flow of available information and may facilitate an overabundance of interchange, curtailing appropriate privacy, or may restrict interaction too severely. Analysis of boundaries between families and larger systems may use the following questions (specifics for the Connors family are in the second column).

What is the usual nature of the family's boundaries with larger systems (i.e., ranging from too diffuse to too rigid)?	Connors family had enduring and diffuse boundary with social services.
What is the usual nature of the larger system's boundaries with families? With other larger systems?	Social Services boundary with families is usually diffuse, and the system anticipates diffuse boundaries with other larger systems.
What is the particular nature of the boundaries between a given family and given larger systems?	Boundary is diffuse between family and eligibility worker, allowing access to information that, in many other families, would remain *in* family; boundary between family and child welfare workers is rigid.
Is there a struggle ensuing regarding appropriate boundaries?	Yes. Family wants to maintain more rigid boundaries with child welfare, who, in turn, is seeking more diffuse boundaries.
Are any of the systems seeking allies in order to renegotiate boundaries indirectly?	Yes. Child welfare is attempting to create alliance with family therapist in order to gain greater access to family.
Is the family–larger system boundary temporary or more permanent?	More permanent, due to family's choice to be foster parents.

Myths and Beliefs

Just as families have myths and beliefs about individual members, specific relationships, and the whole family, which constrain members' views of reality and organize interactions, so families and larger systems have myths and beliefs, regarding one another and their relationships with each other, which either facilitate change or function to maintain the status quo. Myths may be about the other system (e.g., a family's beliefs about larger systems and vice versa) or about the meaning that reflects on one system by virtue of its relationship with the other system. Thus a family may believe that they are a bad family because they are interacting with a larger system. Myths often narrow what families and larger systems are able to see about one another, constrain available relationship options, and contribute to stereotyped cycles of interaction. Thus a family who views a school system with suspicion will focus only on information that supports this belief, often ignoring more positive transactions, while the school whose view of the family is quite negative will not notice when the family is, in fact, supporting its efforts.

It is crucial that the family therapist discern the family's myths about larger systems, lest he or she be quickly painted with the same brush. The family therapist must also detect myths that larger systems hold about the family, in order to avoid adopting beliefs that constrain possibilities for change.

Sources of Myths and Beliefs

A family's larger system myths and beliefs may be part of an intergenerational legacy, may arise out of ongoing experiences, or may result from a critical incident. Here it becomes important to discover if a family is the recipient of strong messages, either implicit or explicit, from extended family and/or its culture regarding larger systems in general or specific larger systems. Like many myths and beliefs from extended family, the myths and beliefs vis-à-vis larger systems are often unexamined by families. Reluctance to engage in therapy, for instance, often becomes explainable when one discovers that key members of an extended family would consider such involvement as proof of craziness. Or a man may carry myths from his family of origin that larger systems are "useless" or "meddlers." A family may carry a legacy of beliefs about specific larger systems, as when parents come from families where involvement with the public school system was uniformly problematic or negative. A family's inherited beliefs about larger systems are often complex, as when parents have differing beliefs inculcated by their families of origin. If a wife comes from a family where people had fairly positive relationships with larger systems and where it was, as it often is, the wife's responsibility to engage with helpers, and the husband comes from a family where larger systems were viewed quite negatively, a helper may easily fall into the trap of seeing her alone, colluding with her despair that her husband won't seek help, and thereby reify intergenerational myths about larger systems.

A family with ongoing relationships with larger systems will often totalize their points of view towards helpers, such that any new helper is quickly defined by the family's agreed-upon myths and treated accordingly.

Sometimes a family may experience a critical incident with a larger system that will be powerful enough to color subsequent involvements. Such critical incidents will be remembered by family members and form the fabric of stories that are repeated. In the family with the daughter who ate only french fries, bread, and milk ("A family born with larger systems"), Mrs. Moore vividly recalled the doctor telling her "don't worry" when her child was born with a heart condition requiring surgical correction. When this incident occurred 12 years earlier, the mother clearly felt disrespected, patronized, and misunderstood at a time when she was frightened and needed both empathy and information. This critical incident formed part of the context of subsequent relationships with larger systems. While such critical incidents are, of course, affected by the family's perceptions of the event and not necessarily a comment on the veracity of the interaction, they are nonetheless crucial to the formation of myths about larger systems.

CASE EXAMPLE (CONTINUED)

The Connors family's myths and beliefs about larger systems arose primarily from its 20-year history with social services. Since workers changed frequently and were often young and inexperienced, the Connorses held the belief that social services *and* other larger systems had little to offer them that would be beneficial. Their lengthy involvement led them to shape the belief about themselves that they were "experts on experts." Any new helper who entered their sphere experienced their scrutiny and judgment and often responded defensively, hence feeding their myths about helpers. Finally, their long history with emotionally distressed foster children contributed to a family myth that they were "saviors of lost children," and this belief made it very difficult for them to reach out for help for their own unit, since to do so equated them in their own minds with their foster children.

The myths and beliefs that larger systems have about families arise from current theories that are passed off as "truth" about human nature, rather than as lenses that make certain information available while proscribing other information; from prejudices about categories of families such as poor families or racial minorities (Lee, 1980); from reports written by other professionals; from information shared at case conferences; and from specific experiences with a given family. Larger systems may also hold myths about other larger systems.

Larger systems often undergo shifts in theoretical perspectives that contribute to rigid beliefs about families. Such theories are presented as the truth and the final word about particular symptoms or situations, despite a paucity of research evidence. From such theories flow definitive working methods. Families that for some reason do not fit the theory are easily categorized via such conceptual myths as "unworkable" or uncooperative. Proffered linear connections, such as "child abusers were frequently abused as children," are uncritically expanded to "anyone abused as a child will abuse his or her own children." The multifaceted richness of any family is easily ignored when theories about *the* incest family or *the* anorexic family are taken as universal truth.

Certain larger systems or specific workers may generate myths from prejudices that totalize their point of view about families. Larger systems are often the carriers of unexamined cultural attitudes towards ethnic minorities, women, and the poor (Imber-Black, 1986d). Other prejudices may be held regarding life-style preferences, kinds of family organization (e.g., single parent), or specific symptoms.

The social service system involved with the Connorses held a general prejudice about all foster families, believing such families were "only doing it for the money." This prejudice precluded noticing behavior in the Connorses or other foster families that would indicate compassion, religiosity, or the desire to care for children.

It is not unusual to find that a school system, whose unspoken mandate is the transmission of middle-class values, has unexamined myths about youngsters and families from middle-class backgrounds and youngsters and families from poor backgrounds. These myths frequently support differential treatment of children who may be presenting very similar behavior but whose families are from different social classes. For instance, a public school referred a wealthy two-parent family for therapy because of the truancy of their 15-year-old son. During assessment, the parents noted that the school had been very cooperative and understanding, had kept them informed all along the way, had previously sent the boy for special testing, and had attempted to counsel him individually. The school was especially concerned, because the boy was "college material."

Another family was referred to family therapy by a probation officer. It was a poor, single-parent family. The presenting problem was truancy by the 15-year-old son, who attended the same school as the first boy, who was truant just as frequently and with the same pattern of spending his days on the streets, and whose family was reported by the school to social services, which engaged the probation department. During assessment, the mother revealed that she had had one unsatisfactory meeting with the school prior to their referral and that no testing or counseling had been given to her son. The school intended to transfer the boy to a vocational school.

The myths and beliefs generated by prejudice may also underpin subsequent referral patterns, as evident in one Canadian community where, for similar behavior, more women were referred to mental health systems and more men were channeled into the legal system.

Larger systems frequently receive ideas about families in the form of reports from other helpers. Such reports are often written as the definitive truth about families and are couched in static, categorical language that neatly omits the interactional or contextual dimension. Individualistic labels abound, describing qualities as if these were inherent to the person or the family. The printed word and the permanency of such reports lend a power far beyond what is appropriate for one person's point of view at one particular point in time. Frequently families are not aware of the content of such reports or the myths generated thereby about them. (See Chapter 5 for a description of family–larger system cocreation of reports.)

Case conferences in which professionals meet to discuss a family may provide another source of myths. When meeting with one's colleagues, it is very easy for a particular viewpoint to be shaped, to the exclusion of other viewpoints. For instance, if several agencies that have been unsuccessful with a family meet, often a focus on the family's deficits will emerge and totalize everyone's point of view, coloring any subsequent interaction with the family. The professionals' own contribution to what is an unfortunate cycle of interaction is often unseen, as the focus remains on the family in isolation from the helping network, in a manner similar to parents discussing a child and omitting their own impact on the child's behavior.

Finally, larger systems may have experiences with a specific family that become the source of the myth. A family may respond angrily to a helper, such as a family with a sick member in the hospital, interacting with a busy nurse, and a myth may be generated that the family is "hostile." No further examination of the source of the anger, such as fear regarding the ill member's future, is considered. Subsequent interactions are placed in the frame of "hostile family," and a self-perpetuating cycle is generated.

CASE EXAMPLE (CONTINUED)

The child-welfare workers involved with the Connors family found the family to be less forthcoming with information about themselves than were other foster families. Hence the myth developed that the family was secretive and so was likely "hiding something." This myth contributed to an interactional cycle in which the social workers attempted to gain more information from the family, the family held back more, and the designation of "secretive" was amplified.

The myths and beliefs that various larger systems hold about each other also affect subsequent interactions with families. Often such myths are generated by one or two unfortunate transactions between larger systems and mitigate against trust, cooperation, or complex future analysis. It is not unusual to hear helpers within one larger system present simple and totalized views about helpers within another larger system (e.g., "All of those nurses at that hospital are . . . ."). Any family interacting with two or more larger systems that hold negative myths about each other is ripe for a process of triangulation.

Interaction of Myths in Families and in Larger Systems

Sometimes the myths that families hold regarding larger systems and the myths that larger systems hold regarding families interact in ways that contribute to difficulties or to no change.

Families and larger systems holding similar myths may participate in an increasingly rigid macrosystem, whose range of options grows more narrow. For instance, if a single-parent family that holds the myth that all single-parent families are inherently weak, broken, and in need of constant larger system involvement meets up with a larger system whose myths about single-parent families are similar, it is likely that a pattern will ensue in which the family "needs" and receives ongoing outside help that never functions to empower the single parent.

Families and larger systems holding conflicting myths may easily generate escalating patterns regarding who knows best.

CASE EXAMPLE (CONTINUED)

In the Connors family–social services macrosystem, conflicting myths were operative. The Connorses viewed themselves in relation to larger systems as "experts on experts," while social services viewed itself in relation to the family as "knowing what's best." Subtle competition for the "expert" designation prevailed. In addition, the Connorses believed they were motivated by a desire to save children, while social services believed they were in it for the money. Such conflicting myths and beliefs underpinned an uneasy relationship marked by mutual suspicion.

Myths regarding the efficacy of professional help in general abound in both families and larger systems and interact in ways that affect any new helping endeavor. Thus, a family may be quite pessimistic about professional help, while the helpers might be quite optimistic, or such optimism/pessimism may adhere to particular families, kinds of problems, or categories of helpers. For instance, a helper may be generally optimistic about the potency of family therapy for most problems, but be quite pessimistic about family therapy for alcohol problems. This belief will, in turn, interact with the family's point of view.

CASE EXAMPLE (CONTINUED)

The larger system was quite optimistic and enthusiastic about the potential of family therapy for the Connors. The family, in turn, was extremely pessimistic about family therapy. Each system worked hard to prove their belief was correct.

The Sociocultural Context of Myths and Beliefs

A common myth pervading the sociocultural context in North America holds that the nuclear family is an independent sanctuary, in need of no outside help or support. This myth forms a potent backdrop for all that occurs between families and larger systems, since families in need of outside help and support—whether from extended family, friends, or professional helpers—often view themselves and are viewed by the helping systems as aberrant. The myth contributes to tension in the macrosystem, and militates against necessary empathy.

Myths and fixed beliefs in families and larger systems about each other and about the meanings of their relationship may constrain the possibilities of generating a complex, multifaceted point of view capable of facilitating change. In addition, such myths and fixed beliefs will affect the entry and subsequent relevance and effectiveness of the family therapist.

The following questions should be asked to determine what myths are involved (specifics for the Connors family are in the second column).

What are the family sources of myths?	There is no obvious intergenerational legacy of myths. A 20-year ongoing history with social services has generated myths that the Connorses are experts on experts and child saviors. There are no obvious critical incidents leading to myths.
What are the sources of myths in the larger systems?	Theories accepted as truth are not discernable in the Connors case. A prejudice exists that foster families only take in children for the money. There is no information on whether reports and case conferences have generated myths. Experience with the Connors family has led the social workers to generate a myth that the family is secretive and withholding information.
In what way are the family myths and the larger systems myths similar?	No similarities are discernible.
In what way are the family and larger system myths in conflict?	The "experts on experts" myth opposes the social services' "we know best" myth. The Connorses' view of themselves as child saviors conflicts with the social

services idea that foster parents are in
it for the money
The Connorses are pessimistic and the
social services optimistic about family
therapy.

Past and Current Solution Behavior

When one works with a family, inquiry regarding attempted solutions are
often part of an initial assessment. One may be seeking to discover the
"more of the same wrong solution" as described by Watzlawick, Weakland, and Fisch (1974) in order to discern behavior or interactional cycles
in the present that are contributing to the ongoing nature of the problem
or symptom, or one may be detecting beliefs that manifest in a narrow
range of behavior, as in a systemic approach that focuses on the family's
world view (Tomm, 1984a, 1984b). Haley (1976) uses a discussion of
solution behavior in order to implicitly highlight previous failures and
thereby motivate the family, as well as to avoid offering "solutions" that
have been tried and found wanting. Finally, a discussion of previous
attempted solutions imparts respect to the family, indicating that the
therapist believes they have been working on the problem and that the
therapist is curious about their ideas and their strengths prior to intervention (Imber-Black, 1986c).

All of the above perspectives on solution behavior come into play
when one is assessing the family–larger system network. The major
difference involves levels of analysis as one becomes interested in the
solutions of families and larger systems, not solely in regard to the
presenting problem but also in regard to one another and in interaction
with one another.

A family's solution to dealing with larger systems may be to always
respond with anger, to refuse access, to lovingly invite helpers in and
absorb them into the family sphere, to pretend to cooperate, to appoint
one member as the person who deals with larger systems, preventing
access to the rest of the family, to engage with larger systems only during
crises, or to interact in ways that split helpers.

Some families are coerced to interact with larger systems, as when
courts order families to treatment. Other families may experience a sense
of powerlessness vis-à-vis helpers, as when a member is very ill and the
family is suddenly required to be involved with the health care system.
Here it is crucial to attend to how the family attempts to solve their
second problem, that of interaction with helpers whom they would often
rather not see at all. Understanding the family's behavior as a solution to
this predicament casts it in a very different light than attributing it to
qualities inherent in the family.

The family's past solutions for dealing with larger systems may be important to discover, as these will often shape what the family believes are its current options.

Larger systems also engage in solutions in regard to their involvement with families. Such solutions may include (1) ignoring family input about problems in an offspring, (2) not including families in plans that are being made, as for instance with a mentally handicapped young adult in a group home setting, (3) overprotecting, patronizing, or feeling sorry for families in ways that reduce a family's own competence to participate in problem solving, (4) becoming a "member of the family" through too frequent interaction, often with one member (Selvini Palazzoli, *et al.*, 1980b), (5) taking on roles that are appropriately within the family's sphere, such as setting rules for a child, (6) utilizing labels that either engender chronicity or hopelessness or require specific treatment that may not fit a family's circumstances, (7) adopting an expert position with families that *never* shifts and ignores family readiness for greater symmetry, and (8) adding more and more helpers and more and more larger systems, thus generating a multiple-helper situation. Larger systems' solutions in regard to families are frequently part of agency policy, treatment philosophy, or informal beliefs. Thus, a larger system may be established within a statutory framework to deliver services to the handicapped. A section of its policy may be to require a client review annually, to which parents are invited. If no other attempts to involve family are made throughout the year, such events are often uncomfortable and tense. Staff may observe that, following weekends home, their client becomes more difficult temporarily, and the informal belief is generated that families make things worse. The solution of avoiding the family or keeping them at a distance grows more rigid and often contributes to the very problem it is meant to solve, as the client misbehaves more in order to get a coordinated message from staff and family or to experience their joint support. In assessing the solutions of the larger system vis-à-vis families, it is important to discern the ideas that underpin such solutions.

A family's solutions regarding larger systems and a larger system's solutions regarding a family will, of course, interact with one another. Often such interaction results in an amplification of preferred solutions. Thus, if a family's solution to a larger system's wishing greater access is to close off more and the larger system's solution in such situations is to attempt to gain greater access or to bring in other larger systems to do so, a vicious cycle will soon emerge. If a family system's solution and a larger system's solution vis-à-vis each other are identical, such as distancing and then growing more suspicious from lack of information, then a macrosystem marked by rigid boundaries and elements of mutual "paranoia" will blossom. If a larger system whose solution is to search after specialists meets a family whose solution is to warmly engage and quickly neutralize each new helper, then a family–multiple-helper system will result.

When the family therapist can discern the solutions of the family in regard to larger systems, he or she can invent ways that challenge the family to create new, more viable solutions vis-à-vis the therapist as representative of a new larger system. Understanding the solutions that other larger systems may have used with the family can enable the therapist to avoid repeating them if they have not been useful and to develop others that may be viable. Conceptualizing those vicious-cycle solutions may provide the therapist with a new level for intervention that includes both family and larger system. (See Chapters 5 and 6 for examples.)

CASE EXAMPLE (CONTINUED)

The Connorses' solutions for dealing with social services included appointing Mrs. Connors as the main conduit to the larger system and protector of the family from larger system intrusion, adopting an air of polite cooperation for any dealings with larger systems, and showing only their successes while minimizing any intrafamily difficulties they might be experiencing.

Social services' solution for dealing with any foster family included periodic review that searched for problems and ignored successes and the involvement of other agencies and other helpers when problems were found or suspected, without first gaining a family's genuine agreement.

The family's and the larger system's solutions interacted in ways that promoted further attempted withdrawal on the part of the family and further attempted intrusion on the part of social services, resulting in a family–multiple-helper system fraught with misunderstandings and suspicion.

Solution behavior in families and larger systems vis-à-vis each other may interact in ways that generate vicious cycles and limit creative and effective solutions. Analysis of solutions may include the following questions (specifics for the Connors family are in the second column).

What are the family's preferred and familiar solutions for dealing with larger systems?	Mrs. Connors acts as conduit to larger systems and gatekeeper for the family. The family cooperates politely and displays only successes.
What are the larger system's preferred and familiar solutions for dealing with families?	Social services holds periodic reviews focusing on problems and uses referrals to multiple helpers.

What are the cycles and outcomes generated when the family's solutions and the larger system's solutions interact?

See Figure 3-3. The cycle has no discernible resolution.

Binds

The communication of two or more simultaneous demands, from families to larger systems and from larger systems to families, that are impossible to meet because they are incompatible may be understood as binds that frequently paralyze effective action. A familiar bind, communicated implicitly or explicitly by a family to larger systems, is "help us to change without changing anything."

Many unintended or unexamined binds are communicated to families from larger systems. Binds in the mixture of messages that a family receives from the wider culture on the one hand and the larger system on the other may be inherent to the practices of particular systems. Thus, there is the ubiquitous bind created by the message from the culture that families are expected to be independent and function without outside assistance, while help-providing larger systems are urging families to receive and accept extrafamilial support. A family may be defined as weak or flawed if they ask for help, while simultaneously being defined as

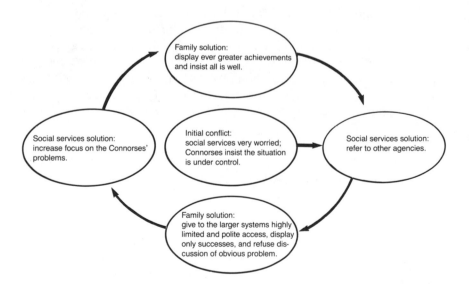

Figure 3-3. The cyclical pattern arising from differences between the Connors family and larger systems regarding problem resolution.

resistant or uncooperative if they refuse help. Larger systems that are part of the legal apparatus (e.g., courts, probation, parole) may create binds by *ordering* families to treatment while simultaneously anticipating that the family will spontaneously *want* treatment and be able to show this despite the coerced context. A bind connected to this and adhering to both legal and welfare systems arises in a macrosystem marked by two incompatible contexts, one of development and trust and one of social control and adverse interests. A family is expected to trust their worker or others to whom they are referred by their worker, while that which they tell their worker may, in fact, be used against them.

Binds may arise in the family–multiple-helper system when the family is referred to more and more helpers, while simultaneously being criticized for overinvolvement in the problem. Conversely, refusal of multiple referrals may lead to a designation of resistant or uncaring.

The relationship between women as mothers and/or single parents and many larger systems is frequently fraught with binds (Imber-Black, 1986d). For instance, a woman who is expected to motivate the rest of her family, particularly her husband, to engage with larger systems may then find herself criticized for this conduit position. The mother may be telephoned weekly by a guidance counselor and then criticized for overinvolvement. She may be encouraged to be dependent on helpers while simultaneously being expected to enter willingly into solutions that stress *only* autonomy and independence for children, ignoring any interdependent options.

A common bind occurs when a family is expected by a larger system to seek treatment and either their compliance or their noncompliance with this expectation is interpreted as evidence of flaws and deficits. The family is damned if it seeks treatment and damned if it does not.

All of the above situations, not surprisingly, lead to unusual behavior as people seek ways to escape the binds.

CASE EXAMPLE (CONTINUED)

The Connors family communicated the familiar "help us to change without changing anything" bind in their request that Alice be "fixed" without changing anything in their family. This bind was fairly apparent. A more subtle bind, however, was that communicated by social services to the family. The Connorses had been a foster family for 20 years without ever being asked to go for therapy. The insistence on therapy now was a message that social services saw them as flawed, and to accept the referral for family therapy was to agree with this assessment and disqualify themselves as a good foster family. On the other hand, if the Connorses refused family therapy they would also be defined as flawed, as they would be seen by social services as resisting help that experts felt they needed. The family's response to this bind was to feign cooperation with the referral, to give minimal information to the family therapist that was just enough to declare they were in therapy but not enough for effective treatment, to go to great lengths elaborating the difficulties of scheduling appointments, and to insist that all of the children made myriad changes after one appointment. This response exacerbated the bind, as social services was sure that they were "protesting too much" in their claims of instant change after one appointment. One can see that if the family reported no changes, that too would be held against them.

A further bind existed because social services expected the family to be open in family therapy and to enter a context of trust, while expecting regular reports from the family therapist, placing family therapy in a supervisory and potentially adversarial context. When the family therapist can discern binds in the family–larger system network, he or she may find unusual behavior more explainable as responses to such binds and be able to intervene to dissolve or otherwise neutralize the binds. (See Chapters 5 and 6 for interventions and full case examples.)

Binds or simultaneous incompatible messages existing in the family–larger system network often curtail effective action and lead to displays of unusual behavior. Such binds are frequently iatrogenic, leading to or exacerbating problematic behavior between the family and larger systems. Analysis of binds may use the following questions (specifics for the Connors family are in the second column).

What binds are the family communicating to the larger systems?

Help us to change without changing anything.

What binds are the larger systems communicating to the family?

You are flawed if you go for treatment and if you refuse treatment.

If you change too rapidly you are pretending; if you don't begin to change you are resisting.

Family therapy is an arena of trust and openness; family therapy will generate reports that will be used to supervise you and may be used against you.

What unusual behavior becomes explainable by reference to binds?

The Connorses feigned cooperation with family therapy while they found it nearly impossible to make appointments.

Minimal sharing of information in family therapy.

Transitions in the Macrosystem

As families and helpers elaborate a macrosystem, transitions requiring changes in rules, roles, and relationships become important to assess. Just as family relationships must undergo profound changes when members enter or exit, so family–larger system relationships must also accommodate such transitions.

For families involved with large public-sector systems, transitions concerning the exit of one helper and the entry of another may breed a certain cynicism, since such changes are frequent and often occur with little or no anticipation. Families may not be told that a worker is leaving, generating a point of view that the role, and not the relationship, is what matters.

Transitions in the macrosystem may also occur via policy changes in the larger systems. Often such changes are not communicated to the families, who begin to experience an unexplained change in their helpers' behavior. For example, some child-welfare departments have undergone policy changes such that a policy of keeping families together has been replaced by a policy of removing children more quickly, which in turn has been replaced by a policy that again focuses on keeping families together. Unless such transitions are demystified for worker and family alike, apathy and mistrust flourishes in the macrosystem.

CASE EXAMPLE (CONTINUED)

The Connors family was used to many transitions, in the comings and goings both of foster children and of social service workers. They had interacted with many, many workers and believed that the relationship between them and any particular worker was extremely temporary. This belief fed their position of simply stalling vis-à-vis the referral for family therapy, since they assumed any given worker would be replaced fairly rapidly.

At the time of their referral for family therapy, the Connorses were not aware of an important policy change occurring in the social service system. After a long period of being encouraged to remove children from their biological families, workers were now being told that they must do whatever they could to maintain children at home and to return children from foster care, wherever possible. The impetus for this transition was fiscal. Workers were urged to examine all of their cases from this perspective and to justify carefully why foster care was preferable to returning children. It was within this context that the referral for family therapy, one aim of which was to scrutinize the foster family, was made.

When a transition in the macrosystem closely matches an unresolved transition in the family, special difficulties may ensue. The loss of a particular helper may be more profound in a family that is struggling to deal with an internal loss. Attending to this issue may allow effective work regarding loss of the helper to be extended metaphorically to internal family losses.

Families who have existed for many years in required, enduring relationships with larger systems may have a difficult time with a transition to being a family without helpers. Thus, the Moores (in "A family born with larger systems") moved immediately from relationships with helpers regarding their daughter's heart condition to relationships with helpers regarding their daughter's eating habits. Change in the family system included a major transition to becoming a family organized without helpers in its sphere. The movement in this transition included a shift from being a family that never questioned or criticized helpers to being a family that felt able to question and criticize helpers and a shift from relying on outside systems to a sense of parental empowerment and appropriate consultation with outside systems.

Transitions in the macrosystem may include frequent entries and exits of helpers, policy changes that are often unknown to families and contribute to mystification, issues of loss that closely mirror family losses, and the need to shift from reliance on helpers to more autonomous functioning. Analysis of transitions may use the following questions (specifics for the Connors family are in the second column).

Is the macrosystem marked by the frequent entry and exit of helpers?	There has been rapid turnover of workers. The family belief is "just wait—a new worker will be along soon."
Are there recent policy changes affecting work in the larger system? Are families cognizant of such changes?	Social services policy changed from heavy use of foster care to reuniting of families, and the Connorses are not aware of the change.
Do transitions in the macrosystem mirror unresolved transitions in the family, especially loss?	Unknown.
Is work needed to effect a transition for the family to function more autonomously?	The Connorses have lived with larger systems in their midst for 20 years; such a transition may be necessary, depending on what occurs regarding their status as a foster family.

Predictions

The final aspect of assessing the family–larger system network regards predictions that the family has about itself and its relationships with larger systems and that the larger systems have about a given family and that family's relationships with larger systems. Secondarily, if one is working only with the larger system, in a consultative format focusing on the system's development, or with two or more larger systems, centering on their relationships with each other, the arena of predictions is also salient.

When families and larger systems describe their imagined futures, especially regarding one another, a family therapist is able to gain access to notions of optimism and pessimism, success and failure, lifelong involvement versus disengagement, and predictions of problems requiring engagement with larger systems.

Predictions feed back into the current macrosystem, as participants behave in ways to support their views of the future. If a family and larger system predict a conflict-filled future, likely they will attend only to those aspects of their relationship that manifest conflict in the present, ignore more peaceful or benign interactions, and amplify the conflict thereby. Likewise, images of a future in which no solutions are found and hopelessness prevails while more and more helpers are added are, without different intervention, likely to yield the predicted result.

When asked to describe their future in regard to larger systems, some families will reveal disappointments or anger with helpers, which they anticipate will continue. Other families will predict finding just the right helper who will solve their predicament, thus making a bid to the family therapist to fulfill this impossible role. Still other families will predict interaction with systems currently outside of their experience, as when parents imagine that their truant son, currently in trouble with the school system, in a year will be in trouble with the legal system. Families who have never been without helpers often find it impossible to envision a more autonomous future and instead predict a multiplicity of new problems that will maintain their relationship to larger systems, even when that relationship is fraught with negativity. Families whose members have a special, warm closeness with helpers, which has either substituted when such closeness is missing in the family or obviated its development in the family, often predict a future that includes continuing problems in the family in order to support the continuance of the special relationship.

When asked to describe the future in regard to particular families, helpers from larger systems may offer ideas that constrain possibilities, as when particular symptoms or problems are predicted to be chronic or lifelong, involving no change, or are seen to interdict variable options. When such predictions fit family predictions, an increasingly narrow range of behavior develops.

Larger system representatives may also predict a particular future based on theoretical beliefs regarding the definitive course of a symptom or set of life circumstances. The predictions of larger systems may be indicative of referral plans previously unknown to the family or the family therapist or may reflect information sent by referral sources or contained in reports or files. If hopelessness is stamped all over the file in various ways, it becomes very difficult for any new helper not to be inducted into this point of view.

Just as families who have warm and special relationships with helpers will predict a future with problems requiring the helper's continued presence, so the helpers will often make similar predictions. But sometimes the image of the future held by the family and that imagined by the helpers differ markedly. Such differences may metaphorically express other conflict in the macrosystem and a struggle regarding who knows best. At other times such differences may indicate a lack of clear exchange of information or the hiding of information known by the larger system, as when a parent whose children have been removed from the home predicts their return while a social worker predicts their maintenance in foster care because he or she knows the requirements for permanency planning, which are unknown by the family. Such differing predictions often lead to escalating conflictual cycles in pursuit of proving one's own view correct.

CASE EXAMPLE (CONTINUED)

When asked, the Connorses predicted that they would continue to be a foster family long after their own children were grown. Further, they predicted, based on their experience, that social workers would continue to change fairly rapidly, so that the family would not be required to follow directives that they did not like. They envisioned future interactions with a larger system that they regarded as fairly impotent.

Social services was far less definite about the Connorses' future as a foster family and predicated such a future on the family's involvement in family therapy. Further, the eligibility worker predicted severe marital problems for Mr. and Mrs. Connors if they would not engage in marital and family therapy.

Two very different views of the future were on a collision course within the arena of family therapy.

Predictions not only inform the family therapist about aspects of the family–larger system relationship but also serve to inform this network about itself, when they are made at a family–larger system interview rather than privately in reports from one helper to another or at case conferences. Predictions place present behavior in a future frame, which often functions as an intervention and provides the family therapist with material to create alternative future scenarios.

Investigating predictions in the family–larger system network often illuminates the nature of relationships in the present while providing areas for intervention in order to alter both present and future. Analysis of predictions may use the following questions (specifics for the Connors family are in the second column).

What are the family's predictions about itself and its relationships with larger systems?	The Connors family will continue as a foster family, thus relating continually with social services. The social workers will have little impact on the family because of frequent changes.
What are the larger system's predictions about a given family and the family's relationship to it or other larger systems?	Social services is uncertain about Mr. and Mrs. Connors' future as foster parents. Their future as a foster family is more likely if the family enters therapy. Marital breakdown is predicted if there is no intervention.
How do the family's and the larger system's predictions fit together?	The predictions are in opposition.

SUMMARY AND CONCLUSIONS

A guide for assessment of the family–larger system relationship includes:

    I. A list of involved larger systems
       A. past
       B. present
    II. Definitions of the problem
       A. agreement/disagreement
       B. larger system mandates
       C. preferred locus of blame
       D. whose problem is it anyway?
       E. hidden agendas
   III. Dyads
       A. complementary
       B. symmetrical
   IV. Triads
       A. detour
       B. cross-system alliance
       C. triangulation
    V. Boundaries
    VI. Myths and beliefs
  VII. Past and current solution behavior

VIII. Binds
   IX. Transitions
    X. Predictions

The elements of assessment may be used in their entirety or in various salient combinations. For instance, one may discover that dyadic patterns and predictions, or triadic patterns, boundaries, and binds, or any other combination of elements, inform a direction for intervention. The assessment is meant to organize information in ways that will be useful to the therapist, the family, and other helpers.

CASE EXAMPLE (CONTINUED)

While this list may make assessment appear lengthy, in fact the assessment material regarding the Connorses was generated during half of the first session with the family and one family–larger system session. As this material emerged, the family therapist was able to avoid myriad traps, including unplanned alliances and splits and accepting a basically tainted referral, while at the same time the Connorses and the social service workers were able to learn a great deal about their relationships to each other. Following this assessment, all agreed that a referral for family therapy was not indicated. Thus an hour and a half of work saved all concerned from the creation of an impossible attempt at a therapy contract. Two months later, Mr. and Mrs. Connors made a private request for marital therapy, separate from their involvement with social services. The Connorses continued as a foster family, as struggles between them and social services were gradually ameliorated.

CHAPTER 4

Interviewing Methods

When one's focus is the family–larger system relationship, three possible interview formats may pertain: (1) interviewing the family about its relationship to larger systems, both historically and currently, without larger system representatives present; (2) interviewing the family and members of the larger systems in the presence of each other; and (3) interviewing delegates from the larger systems about their relationships with the family and/or each other, without family members present. This third format will be discussed in Chapter 8, on consulting to larger systems.

The locus of interest in all three formats is the *relationship* of the family and larger systems and/or among the larger systems. One is searching to clarify the composition of the *meaningful system*, or that configuration of family and larger systems that may be presently functioning in ways that constrain problem resolution and effective development. Covert relationship arrangements and hidden agendas become explicit during such interviews and available for intervention possibilities. The place of larger systems in the family's sphere and the place of families in and among larger systems are illuminated. All of the interview formats initially rely heavily, though not exclusively, on the systemic models' tools of hypothesizing, circular interviewing, and neutrality (Selvini Palazzoli *et al.*, 1980a; Tomm, 1984a, 1984b). As will be demonstrated in Chapter 6, interviews relying on positioning, advocacy, restructuring, and coaching are also utilized, following assessment of the family–larger system configuration. All of the interview formats also potentially constitute interventions by virtue of their introduction of new information into the suprasystem.

INTERVIEWING THE FAMILY ALONE

Interviewing the family alone regarding their perceptions and their experiences with outside systems may occur either early in any therapy, that is, in the first or second session, or as part of ongoing work when family–larger system issues are salient but larger system members are not available to come to sessions for various reasons. (The subject of ongoing work with a family, involving larger system issues, will be addressed in Chapter 5 on interventions and in Chapter 6.) Such interviews are generally conducted by the family's therapist.

In working with any new family (or individual), the therapist devotes a portion of time to discovering who is currently involved with the family and who has been involved in the past. The therapist begins with a brief rationale to the family, indicating that knowledge of their prior and current relationships with outside helpers will facilitate the present work. The therapist, during this initial discussion, should take care to communicate a tone of curiosity and openness and avoid any suggestion of criticism of other helpers, even if the family is critical. The therapist seeks to avoid any unplanned alliances or splits during this information-evoking phase. The therapist is not seeking to criticize these relationships or imply their demise, but rather to assess their potential impact on the family's functioning *and* on the present therapeutic endeavor. In a vein similar to inquiring about extended family, one begins to inquire about involvements with larger systems.

In some cases, this inquiry will last 5 or 10 minutes, as the family indicates that it has no current relationships with larger systems, other than the usual and nonproblematic relationships that many families have with schools and health care systems, and that it has no history of troubled relationships with helpers. The information that no other larger systems have ever been involved, especially with a long-standing problem, may be an indicator of rules against discussing problems with an outsider or may point to secrets with which the current involvement with a larger system will have to deal. Gaining information early on that working with a larger system is an unusual way for a family to approach problems will enable the therapist to mitigate against what might otherwise appear as resistance. In other situations, this inquiry will last the entire session, as the therapist and the family begin to discover the family's patterned embeddedness in larger systems.

Once it is established that the family has other professionals in its sphere or has a history of such relationships, the therapist seeks information regarding the nature of these relationships. Here the therapist is curious about fixed beliefs that may shape the family's relationships to outsiders, critical incidents that loom large in the family members' memories of helpers, patterns of initiating contact with outside systems, alliance patterns, configurations between the family and larger systems that may mirror family interaction, multigenerational involvement with larger systems, attitudes towards specific helpers and specific larger systems, and loyalty issues vis-à-vis particular helpers.

During the process of interviewing the family about larger systems, one is, of course, observing analogic information along with gathering verbal responses. Thus, when a family is discussing various helpers, such indicators as smiles, angry tones, displays of frustration or disgust, rapid subject changes, and so on, enter one's hypothesizing process and serve to shape subsequent questions and directions.

Past Relationships with Larger Systems

When it has been established that the family has a history of relationships with larger systems, whether in reference to the current problem or other problems, one may begin to inquire about the family members' recollections of the relationships. One is not searching for "truth" but for the family members' perceptions that may affect the new helping relationship. Several useful questions are discussed below; while any particular question and its wording must be tailored to the actual family, general categories of questions are available to the therapist.

Who first decided to go for outside help? The answers to this question will immediately illuminate whether the initiation of outside help came from within the nuclear family, as suggested by the extended family or friends, or was the result of influence from larger systems, as when a physician or teacher begins a referral process or a family is coerced by an outside system, such as the welfare department. Whether or not there was family consensus about seeking larger system input will often become obvious at this point.

When one tracks this question through subsequent initiations of contact with larger systems, a specific pattern often emerges. One may see that it is always the father who begins such contacts, or that it is always the mother who is sent or offers herself for outside help, or that the family views itself as having never asked for outside involvement but having received it anyway because of coercion.

This question may also be tracked multigenerationally, enabling the family and therapist to discover, for instance, that in the wife's family, women always initiated contact with larger systems regarding alcohol problems with husbands and sons, while in the husband's family, only men initiated contact with larger systems and then only in extreme crises. The importance of discovering such information is seen in cases where the wife continues to be the conduit to larger systems, as she saw her mother and grandmother do, while the husband refuses to support such contacts, since in his family that was "a man's job" conducted only sparingly. Often the source of such differences has never occurred to the family before, and they have blamed each other and/or helpers for prior failures with larger systems.

BRIEF EXAMPLE: THERAPY MAINTAINS A PATTERN

A divorced couple and their two children were referred to family therapy by another therapist who had seen various configurations of the family for 2 years, without change in a pattern of escalating hostility between the parents. The mother called to set the first appointment. Within half an hour, the father called, angrily demanding to see the new therapist alone first. Prior to therapy even beginning, there appeared to be conflict about initiating contact with a helper. The father agreed to come to one session with everybody. A portion of this session was devoted to exploring the family's relationships with larger systems. When the issue of past initiation of contact with helpers was traced, a pattern emerged in which the children, noticing their mother's sadness, would periodically complain to her about their father. The mother would call the father, who would deny any knowledge of the children's upset, since they had not discussed it with him. The mother would then contact an outside helper and insist that the father come to therapy. He would come with anger and resentment at having been, in his perception, ordered to appear. All family members agreed that the therapist then most often sided with the mother, since the father appeared so resistant. Each failed therapy had reified the parent's negative views of each other. Divorce issues remained unresolved, as intense and unproductive interaction ensued with each new therapy, thus mirroring the old marital relationship.

Of all of the various outside help that your family has had over the years, what did you find was the most helpful? This question can be expanded to examine a continuum from most to least helpful. The question can also be framed to discern whom the family found most helpful, and often the family will focus on specific people, even if the therapist does not initially inquire in this manner.

As family members begin to answer this question, all of their ideas regarding the nature of outside help, the efficacy of particular larger systems, and loyalty to specific helpers, as well as resentments and hostilities, become available. A family may respond that nothing has been helpful, leading one to track their ideas about whether or not help from the outside is ever useful. This may lead to the discovery that the family is waiting for the "perfect" helper, enabling the therapist to raise questions about the viability of the present endeavor. Or one may discover that the family's ideas about what has been helpful run counter to one's usual training, requiring that the therapist stretch his or her assumptions in order to creatively approach the family. One may find that what a particular family member experienced as helpful, others found to be a hindrance. One may then track the usual outcome of such differences in order to plan and implement a more successful relationship.

Beliefs about gender and the nature of family–larger system relationships may also emerge, as one discovers the family's view that, for instance, only men have helped them (or that men have never helped). Such beliefs frequently reflect wider social stereotypes, as in families that will only work with male physicians or that automatically discount female social workers. Most often such information remains covert and hence cannot be transformed into workable issues. Once such material becomes available, many avenues open for effective work.

BRIEF EXAMPLE: A LARGER SYSTEM GHOST

A family with many past and current larger system involvements sought therapy for their 15-year-old son. When asked to come to a family interview, they balked, insisting that the therapist meet alone with the son. Following one such session, the therapist again requested a family session. This time the parents agreed, but at the appointment time only the son appeared. Subsequently, when no progress occurred with the son's violent temper, the parents agreed to come in to discuss their ideas about help. During this interview, an important discovery was made. The father came from a family that had a 25-year relationship with a general practice physician. This man made himself available to the family as a counselor, as well as a physician. His method involved seeing family members individually. The father recalled vivid memories both of being sent to this man when he misbehaved and of seeking him out for all manner of counsel. Clearly, this was the "most helpful" help in the father's experience. The doctor functioned as a parent, grandparent, confidante, friend, ally, and disciplinarian. He served in these roles during the father's boyhood and his early marriage. Thus the wife knew him, too, and utilized him in the same way. The relationship had ended when the doctor died, 10 years earlier. For 10 years the family sought implicitly and unsuccessfully to replace him: each contact with a new helper convinced them further that he could never be replaced, and their loyalty to him simply grew.

This discussion with the family, centering on what had been most helpful in their experience with outside helpers, led to the development of a strategy in which the doctor's memory was evoked and preserved *in the service* of a new different relationship with a larger system. A ritual of mourning was created that enabled the family to honor and respect this special relationship and to feel understood by their new therapist, whom they could now appreciate and with whom they could now work. Deliberate distinctions between the doctor and the new therapist were created, which freed the family from a sense of disloyalty to the beloved doctor and allowed the elaboration of new rules regarding relationships with larger systems. This direction is very different from one that might disparage the past relationship and characterize it as overinvolvement or dependency. Rather, information gathered from the question about prior help was used to generate a new relationship that allowed the family to increase its repertoire of options.

Whom do you think the various involvements with outside systems has helped the most? This question can be expanded to examine a continuum from most to least. It often yields information about alliances between family members and outsiders, as well as shedding light on the issue of problem function, since some problems, apparently belonging to one member, may function to get help, support, or comfort for other members. This question, and variations of it, orients the family to their relational position with larger systems. A family may indicate the belief that their involvement with larger systems has aided no one and that they do not anticipate that such relationships will be efficacious. Family members' beliefs about the capabilities of various outsiders and the systems they represent become available and can inform treatment and referral decisions. In some families, responses to this question will yield an analysis of differences among various larger systems and various family members. For example, a teenage girl may indicate that her probation officer had been most helpful to her father, while the priest had been most helpful to her mother, and that neither had been particularly helpful to her in any overt way. Further inquiry may yield the information that the priest had been the mother's ally and confidante for many years and that the daughter's delinquent behavior functioned to bring home an ally for the father, that is, the probation officer, thus freeing the daughter from her perceived need to occupy this role with the father.

Questions regarding who has been helped sometimes lead to the discovery that the family's belief regarding who needs help has dovetailed with larger system and cultural stereotypes, resulting in an increasingly rigid suprasystem whose range of ideas and options has narrowed by virtue of too much similarity. Thus the wider cultural belief that women are both the most responsible for family relationships and most in need of outside help is often carried unquestioned by various larger systems, creating an unfortunate fit with many families' beliefs.

BRIEF EXAMPLE: MOTHER-BLAME

A two-parent family with an adolescent son had a long history of involvement with a variety of larger systems, including medical systems, public and private schools, psychological services, family therapy, and parent education groups. All of these involvements were ostensibly on behalf of the son, who was failing in school and had a history of poor peer relations. During a discussion of whom the outside systems had helped the most, all agreed that the mother had been helped the most. Questioned further, they indicated the nature of this help as that of support. Further, all agreed, despite the boy's obvious life problems, that the mother needed the most help, and they united in a definition of the mother as overinvolved with her son. Subsequent investigation indicated that all of the helpers also saw the problem as one where the mother needed help in "releasing her son from under her thumb" (a physician's report). In 6 years of involvement with larger systems, no one had framed the problem as, for instance, the father's underinvolvement, the son's lack of responsibility, the parents' needs for teamwork, the school's lack of adequate programs, or a dozen other equally plausible points of view. The mother was never credited for dedication but was criticized for a situation supported by the culture and multidetermined by all family members and the helpers. The family's and the larger systems' viewpoint, that the mother needed help to change, converged, resulting in no new options and simply cycling and recycling a pattern in which the mother, sent by the father for help or called in by helpers, was then criticized by both family and helpers for being overinvolved, while the father was working at his career 60 hours a week.

What has your mother (father, other extended family, ex-spouse, etc.) thought about your working with professionals on this issue? Have they favored it or not? Have they thought the outside helpers were helpful or not?

This set of questions links the nuclear family, the extended family, and larger systems and illuminates crucial connections regarding loyalty, multigenerational myths about larger systems, and ethnic and cultural responses to larger systems. In a two-parent family, differences emerge in messages coming from the wife's family about larger systems and those coming from the husband's family.

A family may respond that they are keeping their involvements with larger systems a secret from extended family. Or they may indicate that the wife's family knows and approves of the helping endeavor but that it is a secret from the husband's family, whom they are certain would disapprove. Such secrets are important indicators of loyalty issues regarding extended family. One may discover that family members are supposed to turn to a particular member, either for help or for permission to seek outside help, yet have kept the entire endeavor a secret. Secrets function as boundary markers, defining who is "in" in a particular relationship and who is "out." Such secrets regarding larger systems often represent an attempt to gain autonomy, gone awry because the family or individuals may remain tied via a fear of criticism, should extended family discover the relationship with helpers. Secrets regarding relationships with outside helpers may also be metaphors for other secrets between the family and extended family and can be tracked as such. One can make effective use of hypothetical questions regarding the effects of opening the secret and, with the family, can discover intricacies of relationships between the family, extended family, and larger systems.

Information becomes available, that some extended family members disparage either outside help or particular larger systems. It is important that the therapist not be critical or unwittingly enter triangles. Rather, one seeks to explore what the family knows about the basis for these beliefs. Often, unfortunate past experiences with helpers or cultural and ethnic patterns regarding family privacy are at the core of a stance against engagement with outside systems.

Discussion of the extended family's point of view towards larger systems opens many areas for inquiry and intervention, as the family begins to experience itself in multiple, embedded contexts. One may discover with the family, for instance, that the husband's family of origin is quite negative towards professional helpers because they believe help failed them when a member committed suicide. Subsequent family–larger system endeavors will exist in a context of anger and expected failure, unless one works to explore this level and create a relationship that is unanticipated. One may find that the views of different extended family members towards the presenting problem are perfectly replicated by multiple helpers (see the case "A family born with larger systems," Chapter 2), thus reifying patterns at various levels.

Forming relationships with larger systems at various points in the family life cycle may be part of an extended family tradition, as is often seen in families with multigenerational problems with alcohol (Miller, 1983). As one's focus changes from the present family and its alcoholic member to the family's and extended family's past and present relationships with larger systems regarding the problem, a host of new intervention possibilities that do not replicate prior failed attempts become available.

BRIEF EXAMPLE: DEFINING "PIONEERS"

A severely conflicted couple had three unsuccessful attempts at marital therapy in 2 years. They were embarking on their fourth attempt as one last try, indicating to the therapist that if this did not work, they would divorce. The therapist devoted a portion of the interview to examining prior help and began to focus on the extended families' points of view towards these efforts in particular, and towards larger systems in general. Some very important information, never before covered, emerged. The husband's parents, who were Jewish, immigrated to Canada from Morocco. Their experiences with larger systems were generally filled with fear, and they embraced the belief in Canada that one should stay as far away as possible from larger systems. The husband kept all of the couple's attempts at therapy a secret from his parents. One of the wife's major complaints about the husband was that he had participated reluctantly in the prior therapies, but she had always viewed this as a message to her regarding his refusal to participate fully in attempts to save their marriage, rather than viewing him as unwittingly caught between her and his parents, regarding the issue of outside systems. The wife came from a Roman Catholic family. When she was a child, her family had many involvements with larger systems, because of her father's alcoholism. While these interactions were generally nonproductive, nonetheless interaction with larger systems regarding family problems was a familiar legacy, and her mother knew and heartily approved of the couple's interactions with helpers. The husband had converted when he married, and while this issue had been thoroughly explored in the other therapies, the couple's loyalties to their families of origin, as demonstrated through their unsuccessful relationships with helpers, had not been explored until a fourth and final attempt at therapy. Once the intricate relationships of the couple, their extended families, and the larger system came into full relief, distinctions could be drawn among the husband's family's experiences in Morocco with larger systems, the wife's family's experiences with larger systems regarding her father's drinking, and the current therapeutic endeavor. Questions regarding "permission to succeed" with a larger system were framed and functioned to draw the couple together as a unit in their own right. The couple was defined as "pioneers" in creating a new and positive relationship with the outside world via the therapeutic system, and a ritual was implemented to free them from old, no longer viable messages regarding relationships with larger systems.

What do you think various representatives of larger systems have thought of your family? What might these people tell me about working with you? What might their advice be to me? Would you agree or not agree with this advice? How do you think these people might compare you to other families they have worked with?

This series of questions and those to which they idiosyncratically lead begin to inform both therapist and family about the family's perceived experiences with larger systems, as well as their fantasies.

Differences that the family draws among various helpers and larger systems become available, as for instance when family members reply that Mrs. Smith, from child welfare, thought poorly of them, while Mr. Atlas, from probation, thought well of them. Alliances between particular family members and particular helpers are also illuminated with this set of questions, as family members begin to draw distinctions regarding larger system representatives' points of view towards various family members.

Questions regarding what advice family members think past helpers would give the new therapist place the family in the intriguing position of momentary observers and commentators on themselves in relationship to larger systems and as temporary consultants to the new therapist. From this position, family members often let the new therapist know precisely what is needed to engage in an effective manner, without replicating prior failures.

Whether the family has had highly adversarial experiences with helpers, relationships in which they felt criticized, warm and cozy interactions, or highly productive relationships with larger systems becomes quite clear with these questions.

Many families give outside professionals tremendous powers of definition, and shape their image of themselves by what they perceive they have been told by larger systems. Most often this is an implicit process, not examined or questioned until an interview focuses on and challenges such ideas. If the family has seen negative reports written about them, often the power of the written word will nail down the family's image of itself as reflected by outsiders. The questions suggested here can be used both to generate information *and* to cast doubt on reified viewpoints.

BRIEF EXAMPLE: A "BAD" FAMILY

A session was held with a family whose oldest child, a boy, was living in a group home. The family consisted of a mother and a father and two adopted children, ages 8 and 11. The mother was an immigrant from Eastern Europe. The family had lots of prior experience with larger systems, commencing with the adoption home studies and continuing when it was discovered that the boy had both health and learning problems. Through messages from the extended family that were negative about adoption, the parents considered themselves "not good," unable to give birth to children of their own. In response to questions about what the parents thought the various helpers thought of them, their perception was the same over and over again—larger systems thought they were a bad family, incapable of properly raising their children. Final evidence for this came in the boy's removal, as the mother said, "They wouldn't have removed him if they thought we were a good family." They cited examples of criticisms from helpers, which they did not balk at but felt they deserved. The tone of the interview was one of self-effacement and shame. The family's view of itself fit what they *perceived* outsiders' views to be and went unchallenged until this interview, feeding a cycle that resulted in the boy's placement in a group home. Detailed exploration of what the family thought helpers thought of them revealed a picture in which the parents, already unsure and down on themselves, became the recipient of lots of advice about how to be better parents, which they experienced as appropriate criticism of them. The mother's uncertainty, which she openly showed to helpers, since she was eager to be a good mother, resulted in more and more advice, which simply fed her unsureness with her son, who escalated his behavior, sending her to the next helper. A focus on what the family thought helpers thought of them illuminated this pattern and enabled the new therapist to develop a strategy that focused on hidden strengths of the family, reframing their experiences with critical helpers as evidence of their resources, endurance, and strengths.

Exploration of Critical Incidents

As the family responds to the various questions discussed above, a focus on particular critical incidents between the family and larger systems often emerges. Such critical incidents may shape and affect all subsequent interactions with larger systems, form the core of the family's beliefs about helpers, and create an unexamined context within which each new helping endeavor exists. Often such critical incidents occur at nodal family life-cycle transition points, such as marriage, the birth of children, divorce, leaving home, the onset of serious illness, and so on, such that the life-cycle events and interactions with larger systems become intertwined. An initial critical incident may be replicated, both by accident and by selective design. Any new therapist entering the family sphere needs to know about critical incidents between the family and larger systems, in order to fashion a new relationship that may be capable of recontextualizing old beliefs.

BRIEF EXAMPLE: A "DOOMED" MARRIAGE

A couple married for 14 years embarked on marital therapy. Six sessions were held, during which the therapist discovered that the couple was quite isolated and had no support from family or friends. The wife had been pregnant when the couple married, and their families of origin were angry and critical. A pattern of the couple virulently criticizing each other appeared unamenable to change. In the sixth session, the couple also began to criticize the therapist for being unable to help them, "just like all the others." As this was the first mention of others and since therapy appeared stuck, the therapist sought supervision. At the presession, the therapist's obvious frustration with the case was expressed as criticism of the couple. It was decided to explore the couple's relationship to these unnamed others.

During the session, focusing on the couple's experience with helpers, the wife related that she went to a psychiatrist soon after they married because she felt so unhappy. Queried regarding her recollection of this experience, she stated that he told her, "Too bad you didn't come in before you got pregnant!" She could remember little else and said she interpreted this to mean that their marriage was doomed from the start. This interpretation was exacerbated by the first psychiatrist referring her to a colleague after only one session, which she took to mean that their situation was hopeless. Asked to describe this relationship, she said, "He helped me along until I was able to deliver. I leaned on him, but he also taught me that leaning on someone is an illness." Any desire she had to use her husband for support was interdicted. During her therapy, the husband also saw a therapist. His recollection of this experience was that the therapist's advice was "go find yourself another girl." He also took this to mean that his marriage was doomed. During the years of their marriage, the couple related various attempts at seeking therapy, all of which ended in frustration and increased despair. One marriage counselor "washed his hands of us after four sessions." What was striking in listening to the couple was their highly selective recollections of therapies. Beginning with the first therapy, which occurred at the life-cycle transition to a marriage that already existed in a context of criticism, the couple, individually and collectively, found and exquisitely remembered criticism from the various helpers. A cycle, marked by the couple criticizing each other, finding helpers who they felt criticized their marriage, which in turn led to further criticism of each other, continued without end. Any new helping endeavor existed in this context of doom. The couple did not consider divorce, stating that this would prove their parents right. Curiously, divorce might also prove the various helpers "right," although the couple did not acknowledge this. This interview freed the current therapist from any propensity to criticize the couple and replicate the prior pattern. Interventions were designed to make use of the definition "doomed marriage" in paradoxical ways, and the couple was given a ritual to "rewrite their history" with larger systems (see Chapter 5 for an elaboration of this type of intervention), such that the reification of doomed marriage could be challenged. A successful therapy ensued.

The above example highlights the need to examine critical incidents between the family and larger systems. It is important to remember that one is not seeking the truth regarding the family–larger system relationship, but the family's recollected metaphors and stories that form a backdrop for any new family–larger system relationship. Usually the family will describe critical incidents with a high degree of affective expression, recalling key phrases and emotions. Such critical incidents form the core of a family's myths about larger systems. As such, they need to be explored and utilized.

Present Relationships with Larger Systems

Many of the questions cited above may, of course, be tailored to explore current relationships with larger systems. Thus, one may wish to explore what or whom is presently most helpful and to whom, current extended-family ideas about larger systems, and what family members think present helpers think of them now. In addition to these areas, however, one is especially interested in the family's experience of the referral process and their ideas about ongoing relationships with larger systems.

What are your ideas about why the physician (school counselor, social worker, therapists, minister, etc.) suggested that you come here? Or insisted that you come here? Who is most in favor of this referral?

These questions may indicate that the family feel they were ordered to therapy and have no choice about who the therapist is, that the family are confused about the referral since they experienced their work with the referring person as going well, or that one member is especially pleased with a new opportunity, while the others are diffident. Information may emerge that one family member has a special, ongoing relationship with a referring person (Selvini Palazzoli *et al.*, 1980b) and expects to maintain this relationship, regardless of what happens in the current therapeutic endeavor. Or one may discover that the new therapy was presented to the family as *the* answer, often raising expectations that cannot realistically be met. Finally, one may find that two or more referrals for similar services have been made simultaneously, immediately generating a family–multiple-helpers system.

BRIEF EXAMPLE: WHY ARE WE HERE?

A family consisting of two parents and two children, ages 10 and 12, was referred to family therapy by a woman who had been working with the couple for over a year. The family came haltingly to the new therapist. After five sessions with no progress, a consultation was arranged. During this consulting interview, in response to the above questions, the family expressed great confusion about the referral per se, stating that they had liked the other therapist very much and that they were coming to the new therapist because they had been told they had family problems and their prior therapist did not see children. The parents felt both rejected by and loyal to their first therapist, and these feelings permeated the new therapeutic endeavor. Further, the mother stated that she continued to call the first therapist at least weekly, and that their discussions focused on the current therapy. Thus the present family therapy existed in an enduring context that included the prior therapist. From this discovery, plans were made to hold an interview that included the first therapist, in order to effectively delineate boundaries and to develop a viable treatment context.

Many families require ongoing relationships with larger systems because of members with physically and/or mentally handicapping conditions. Several questions may be useful to understand and effectively utilize such relationships.

What do you understand the various larger systems' and helpers' definitions of your problem to be? Are there disagreements over definitions between the family and larger systems or among the various larger systems? What helper is responsible for what aspect of the situation? To whom do you turn in emergencies or crises?

Utilizing these questions, one may discover fixed beliefs regarding the specific nature of chronicity that omit any idiosyncratic development, or one may discover that the family is confused by splits among the larger systems' beliefs and actions, that the family is bewildered regarding the delineation of specific responsibilities, or that the family always turns to one favorite person who responds even when the response is beyond the definition of his or her job.

BRIEF EXAMPLE: HANDICAPPED BY MULTIPLE HELPERS

A single-parent mother, Ms. Hart, had one child, a 10-year-old son, who had been diagnosed as severely retarded. The father left the family, moved away, and remarried shortly after the child's birth, and while he sent support payments and had intermittent contact with the boy, his position was that the mother was the best care-giver and that he could not take his son for visits. At the same time, he encouraged his former wife to place the boy in a group home for mentally handicapped children.

The mother was a competent legal secretary. Her work outside the home had required her to rely on a variety of child-care providers over the years.

Ms. Hart's family-of-origin escaped Europe in 1940. They refused to acknowledge the child's handicaps. They visited infrequently. When the mother tried to discuss her situation and her need to make decisions regarding her son, all of her extended family changed the subject or otherwise minimized her concerns. She reflected often that Hitler killed all mentally handicapped people, believed that such attitudes were still quite rampant, though more underground, and saw her role as a protector for her son. In this regard she had chosen to have no social life and to devote all her nonemployment hours to her child. Her most intense adult social interaction was with professional helpers, who talked with her not only about her son, but also about her life, and filled roles usually held by friends and family.

Because of her son's situation, Ms. Hart had to interact with several larger systems, including her son's school, where she was involved with two special education teachers, a counselor, a speech therapist, and a psychologist; a specialized day care where her son went after school; a government agency involved with mentally handicapped children, which provided her with a caseworker whose job was to coordinate services; and a children's hospital's developmental disability clinic. Because she was required to attend many day-time appointments, she had lost two prior jobs. Her present employer was quite reasonable and allowed her to use a flex-time approach to her work.

Ms. Hart described feeling a lot of tension regarding daily and long-term decisions for her son, as a result of advice she received from larger systems. For instance, the school psychologist urged her to quit her job in order to spend more time with her son, while her caseworker insisted that work outside the home benefited both Ms. Hart and her son. Indeed, the caseworker urged her to utilize weekend group home services as respite care, while still other professionals warned her that such services were not adequate. Predictions regarding her son that were made by the various professionals were confusing and contradictory, ranging from institutionalization at the one remaining large institution for the handicapped, to group home living and a sheltered workshop, to remaining with his mother. Not surprisingly, Ms. Hart's thoughts became paralyzed when she attempted to view the future. Without an understanding of the complex context in which Ms. Hart was embedded, therapeutic endeavors with her would be impossible.

A therapist working with Ms. Hart, or others with similar situations, must appreciate the requirement for ongoing interaction with larger systems, the stress often generated thereby, and the need to intervene in ways that promote autonomy, enhance family resources, and facilitate empowerment of the family on behalf of their handicapped member.

Future Relationships with Larger Systems

Families with past and/or present relationships with larger systems often have ideas regarding the future of these relationships. Such future scenarios span a continuum from hope to despair. They may include keeping a problem in order to maintain a particular helper. They may highlight that a family envisions a future without larger systems, or that a family can envision no future that differs in any way from its present involvement with larger systems. The therapist's task is to gather information regarding the family's view of its future relationships with larger systems.

What do you imagine the family's relationship with social services (the hospital, probation, etc.) will be like in a year? In 5 years? If this present problem is solved, what will happen between [specific family member] and [specific helper]? Will [specific family member] need outside help in a year? In 5 years?

Such questions often shed light on ways that a problem functions at multiple levels of the macrosystem, on alliances between specific family members and specific helpers, and on rigid views of the future described as no different from the present.

BRIEF EXAMPLE: SHE'LL BE FINE IN 5 YEARS

A family consisting of two parents and three teenage children was engaged with multiple helpers, including a family therapist, a probation officer, an alcohol program worker, and an individual therapist. All had entered the family's sphere in the prior year because of delinquent behavior of the oldest child, a girl, 16. Helpers entered primarily at the request of the probation officer and secondarily at the request of the father. The daughter generally refused to cooperate with the various helping endeavors. During a portion of the interview devoted to views of the future, every family member agreed that the daughter would be fine in 5 years and that she would have a successful life. More strikingly, in this system in which more and more helpers were entering, all agreed that she would change her behavior *without* professional help and that the present involvement of helpers made her more stubborn. The revelation of this future scenario led to exploration of the fact that the family's purpose for the helpers was different from what the helpers thought. Indeed, the parents had a deeply troubled marriage and felt unable to ask for appropriate help, since they feared this meant they were failures. Each had covertly hoped that helpers, ostensibly for the girl, would somehow discover and assist with their marital problems. Following this exploration of their views of the future for the identified patient and her relationship with helpers, a more direct marital therapy contract was negotiated, and the girl's behavior improved dramatically.

After one gathers the family's ideas about their future relationships with larger systems, one may be able to pose hypothetical questions that challenge the family's viewpoint and introduce previously unconsidered ideas. Variations of such questions may include: Suppose [specific helper] were no longer available to you—what do you think would happen? What if the family existed without any larger system involvement for 6 months—what would happen to the family (specific family members, the presenting problem, specific relationships)? Suppose your grandmother did find out that you were seeing therapists—what might happen to your relationship with her, to your relationship to the therapists?

All manner of hypothetical scenarios may thus be posed to the family, focusing on the family–larger system relationship.

BRIEF EXAMPLE: LET'S YOU AND HIM FIGHT

During a family interview, lots of information was generated indicating a lengthy past conflictual involvement with multiple helpers and an intense, conflictual present involvement with two helpers, a physician and a social worker. In addition to conflict between the family and the larger systems, the physician and the social worker, representing a children's hospital and social services respectively, also quarreled with each other. When asked about the future, the family members responded with a vision of continued conflict between the family and larger systems and among the larger systems. No sense of an alternate future appeared available. The therapist then posed a question regarding the family's ideas about their future relationship with him. At first they began to describe imagined future conflict with a therapist they had just met. As the absurdity of this scenario emerged, all fell silent. The therapist then posed a hypothetical question that envisioned future cooperative relationships in the macrosystem. "What would happen regarding your son's problem if everyone could agree on a course of action?" What emerged was the family's belief that the parents would then quarrel with each other on many other matters that were neatly submerged by the pattern of conflict in the macrosystem. Work could then focus on this salient issue.

Interviewing the family about its relationships with larger systems is most usefully done in a first or second interview, although the issue may be addressed in later interviews as well, especially if therapy appears stuck for unknown reasons. Therapeutic impasses often result from problematic family–larger system relationships. Such interviewing may be divided along temporal lines, exploring the family's past, present, and imagined future relationships with larger systems. All of the purposes of assessment described in Chapter 3 are intended by such an interview. In addition, based on information generated regarding family–larger system relationships, a therapist may decide that a joint family and larger system interview would be beneficial.

INTERVIEWING THE FAMILY AND LARGER SYSTEM REPRESENTATIVES

There are two points during an ongoing therapy when a family–larger system interview may be appropriate and effective. The first is early on in a case when one discerns that a family is engaged with multiple helpers. The purpose of such an interview is generally to clarify roles and expectations among the family members and helpers. If the family has a long-standing relationship with one or more of the helpers, then patterns and themes may also be addressed. Such an interview is particularly useful if there seems to be confusion regarding the intention of a referral, if the referral is statutory (e.g., a family is ordered to therapy by a court), or if the referral is quasi-statutory (e.g., a family experiences itself as coerced into therapy by a welfare department or a school).

The second useful time for a family–larger system interview is when ongoing therapy has reached an impasse. The therapy may be proceeding with little or no progress, or earlier progress may not be maintained. If the family is presently engaged with larger systems, then a consulting interview should be arranged to include the family and as many of the appropriate larger system representatives as possible. The purpose of this interview is to elicit patterns and themes in the suprasystem, to inform the suprasystem about itself, and to design and implement effective interventions to achieve therapeutic goals. The purpose is decidedly *not* to direct the multiple helpers or to tell them how to do their jobs, since there is no contract to do so and such actions only engender resentment in the larger systems.

The Role of the Consultant

When a family–larger system interview is held, it should be conducted by a consultant rather than by the family's therapist. Since the family therapist is part of the family–larger system network, his or her position in the suprasystem should be assessed along with the other members'. In addition, professionals involved in a case tend to define their relationships with one another as symmetrical, and so may feel put down if the family therapist conducts the interview. The possibilities of eliciting cooperation are greater in a consultant-facilitated interview.

The consultant's job is to inquire about the system formed by the family and larger systems and to offer opinions and ideas in order to introduce new and usable information to the suprasystem. No one is expected to be held accountable to the consultant in this context, and no effort should be made by the consultant to direct people's work back in their own settings. Thus the consultant should not be the family therapist's supervisor. Colleagues who are well versed in systemic thought and practice can effectively function in the consulting role. Following the interview and any interventions that are made, the consultant must take care to exit from the case and not become yet another member of the suprasystem.

Inviting the Participants

When a family–larger system interview is held with a consultant, it is the family's therapist who invites the participants. The meeting should be organized at a time that is convenient for as many as possible. It is important that the scheduling constraints of the various larger system representatives be respected if cooperation is to be achieved initially (e.g., physicians often require early morning meetings; school personnel often require early morning or late afternoon meetings). A family–larger system meeting can easily get off on the wrong foot if scheduling requests by the participants are immediately framed as resistance rather than as information about the demands of each system, as translated by a particular participant. Matching the schedules of the family members, the helpers, and the consultant can sometimes be difficult work, but if short shrift is given to any of the participants' stated needs in this area, a tone of disrespect may be set.

In the invitation to the participants, the therapist should make it clear that this is a consultation that he or she is seeking in order to enhance his or her work with the family. The same use of joining skills that one uses to invite family members to a first interview should be utilized. Care should be taken in order to not communicate blame, criticism, or any aura of extrusion to the larger system representatives. In asking the participants' assistance in this endeavor, the therapist may also frame the occasion as an opportunity for the family–larger system network to learn about itself, enabling the possibilities of new decisions based on new information. The sheer act of inviting the family and helpers to such a meeting is an intervention in the macrosystem, as the invitation implies often previously unseen connectedness. The meeting per se is "news of a difference," as families and multiple helpers rarely, if ever, sit down together. An intervention in previous fragmentation and in the often complementary relationship of clients and helpers is made when all agree to come to the consultation and share ideas, plans, and information openly.

Occasionally, a larger system member will not come to the meeting, because of the high degree of anger in the macrosystem or a wish to distance and not be involved, because a supervisor refused permission, because of a fear of vulnerability, or because of a straightforward scheduling conflict (e.g., a welfare worker called to the court at the last moment). Care should be taken not to criticize or scapegoat this person or to forget about the person's place in the macrosystem. Information generated in the interview should be communicated to such absent members, unless it has been clarified that they are no longer part of the meaningful system.

Format and Focus of the Interview

A presession is held with the consultant, the therapist seeking the consultation, and any team members who may be working with the consultant. Invited professionals from the larger systems may ask to meet with the consultant prior to the family–larger system interview. It is usually best to honor such requests by asking them into the presession, since not to do so may generate resentment and a fear of secrets. After gaining sufficient background regarding the course of the therapy and larger system involvement, the consultant and any team members may meet briefly without the therapist or any other professionals from the macrosystem, in order to hypothesize and plan the initial stage of the interview.

During the interview the consultant's questions focus on the macrosystem formed by family and helpers. The consultant does not delve into family issues per se, except as these interact with the family–larger system relationships. For instance, there may be questions about the family-of-origin experience with and views of helpers but not about other family-of-origin issues. To investigate specific family issues is the job of the family therapist. Also, the consultant needs to be sensitive to boundaries between the family and helpers and to protecting the family's privacy. A family may have discussed marital conflict with their therapist but not with a school teacher who is attending the family–larger system interview. Knowledge of such marital conflict may be outside the appropriate purview of the school personnel and thus should not be raised by the consultant. Rather, the consultant is curious about alliance patterns in the macrosystem, competing beliefs regarding the presenting problem and its etiology, preferred locus of blame, appropriate or optimal solutions, views of the future, and so on.

When the session begins, the consultant should immediately attend to the map of relations that may be communicated analogically by seating arrangements. Alliances may be made apparent by specific family members and helpers sitting next to each other or by several helpers sitting around one family member, while other family members group together. When anger and hostility marks the family–larger system relationship, it is not unusual to see the family sit on one side of the room, while the larger system representatives sit on the other.

Occasionally, the analogic messages may be more blatant, as when helpers and family members touch each other fondly or make significant eye contact. The following are two examples of this kind of message.

1. In a session involving several helpers and a family of two parents and an adolescent girl, the girl sat far from her parents, between a foster mother and a youth counselor, each of whom held her hands and patted her frequently, while the parents sat between their marital therapist and their minister.

2. In a session involving two parents and their three children, the father answered all of the consultant's questions while gazing at his individual therapist. In turn, the therapist looked only at the father when he was speaking. The strength of this alliance, hypothesized from the analogic information, was borne out by other family members' comments.

The various seating arrangements and other analogic communication contribute to the consultant's relational hypotheses to be explored during the interview.

The consultant generally begins by thanking everyone for coming and by orienting the participants to the purpose of the interview. It is important that the consultant reclarify his or her role.

CONSULTANT: I've been asked by the family therapist to consult regarding the Smith family with whom you are all involved. I'm not here to tell anyone how to do their work. Rather, in our experience with families who are engaged with more than one outside helper, we often find it useful to get everyone together in order to clarify roles, expectations, decisions, and so on. If I come up with any new ideas this morning, these will be shared with all of you.

Thus a tone of respect and openness is set in the beginning moments of the interview. At the same time, a rather unusual proposition is being suggested, namely, that family members and helpers will be privy to the same information, temporarily altering the usual helper–helpee complementarity. Such a shift implicitly raises the possibility of new patterns in the macrosystem.

Defining the Roles and Problems

Initial questions are generally role related. The consultant queries the various participants from the larger systems regarding their jobs in general, their specific roles with this family, and the mandate of their larger system. During this portion of the interview, the consultant is being educated regarding the various larger systems. It is not unusual for the family members and the various helpers also to be learning new information about the different larger systems. While this portion of the interview often sounds quite straightforward and factual, it can be an intervention in the boundaries of the components of the macro-system.

Several key factors may emerge during this portion of the interview.

1. Family members may express that they were not aware of the particular roles of certain helpers. Services that they are entitled to may become clearer.

2. Alliance patterns may begin to emerge as a helper indicates his or her usual job role differs in particular ways from what he or she does with a member of this family. Often this difference involves spending far more time with the family member or on the family member's behalf, or performing functions that are unusual. For instance, one may hear a school guidance counselor describing his usual job with the children. As the consultant begins to inquire how his work is the same or different with this family, the counselor may begin to describe how, in this case, he frequently stops at the home and discusses the child with the mother over coffee.

3. Previous unspoken or implicit conflicts among the various larger systems' mandates may begin to emerge in this portion of the interview. Systems whose work is at cross-purposes or whose mandates contradict each other can often confuse or overload a family with conflicting input. Seldom do the representatives of such larger systems have an opportunity to sit down together with family members, in an atmosphere of mutual respect, in order to examine these differences and hear how a family is experiencing being the recipient of contradictory ideas or services. Here the consultant's questions are directed at eliciting the differences and the family's responses to them, without making overt judgments of right and wrong. This is an early portion of the interview, when one is most interested in generating information and tracking emerging patterns and themes.

4. Duplication of services may become apparent. For instance, it is not unusual for participants to discover that a family therapist and a probation officer both see their appropriate role as meeting with the parents to discuss child management and marital issues.

Next the consultant asks for everyone's ideas about definitions of the problem or problems that bring the family and helpers together, ideas about the best approaches to work on the problem, and current views of how such work is going. Patterns of agreement or disagreement, wide divergences of opinion, alliances, and splits generally emerge. If a family is considered multiproblem by the various helpers, then one will usually hear about specialities whose work may or may not be in conflict. Family members may describe that they very much like having different people work on various problems, or they may state that they find it all very confusing. It may be discovered that what the family considers most important is not what the helpers consider most important. One may also find during this portion of the interview that the helpers are far more concerned about particular work being done than the family is. Varying agendas for change or no change often become clear.

Emergence of Themes and Patterns

During the early portions of the interview the consultant is beginning to hypothesize about patterns and themes that seem to mark the macrosystem. Subsequent questions and discussion during the interview are fashioned from these hypotheses and feedback from the participants. All of the questions used when interviewing the family alone about its relationships to larger systems are again useful at this juncture. It is often very enlightening for the various helpers to hear the family describe their past experiences with helpers and to begin to see their own work with the family as existing in a historical context of frequently replicated patterns and themes. It is not unusual for a new helper joining the macrosystem to discover that he or she is one of a long line of helpers who have been initially greeted with great enthusiasm, followed by subsequent disillusionment. Often helpers are finding out for the first time that their helping endeavor exists in a context of rules from families of origin, regarding the correctness and efficacy of outside help.

Discussion of past help is generally followed by more in-depth exploration of the present relationship between the family and helpers. Areas for discussion include patterns of contact, purposes of the current helping endeavor, optimism/pessimism, and comparisons.

Patterns of contact. The consultant is interested in who talks to whom about what. Often in complex family–larger system interactions, only certain people are privy to certain information, while others remain ignorant of plans and actions until after the fact. Such alliance patterns may be between particular helpers, but often they are between specific family members and specific helpers. Thus, a mother and a physician may speak frequently about other family members and other helpers, without such information being relayed to the interested parties. Or one family member may see a helper, while others refuse to go but may be informed about the sessions, thus using this member as a conduit to the larger systems. Family members may discover that various helpers are discussing them without their knowledge, as when a number of personnel from one system become involved in a case. Generally such patterns of contact are not known in the macrosystem until this consultation. This open discussion generally effects subsequent patterns of contact, as the consultant gently challenges boundaries that are either too rigid or too permeable.

Purposes of the current helping endeavor. While definitions of the problem have been discussed earlier, often there are additional reasons why people are getting together that have not been stated. Such hidden agendas of the family and the larger systems may become available in a number of ways. One may ask questions regarding who people think has been helped the most. It is not unusual to find that this is not the person for whom the help is ostensibly intended. Here implicit beliefs about blame and locus of responsibility may emerge, as when family members and helpers agree that the mother has been helped the most to become less involved.

Another purpose of the current helping endeavor that may emerge is the expectation by one larger system that another larger system is going to find out information for them. One may also discover that people had certain unspoken purposes in mind when particular referrals were made but that these purposes were never made explicit. This may include the cynical purpose of expecting failure where others have failed.

Optimism/pessimism. Questions about purposes lead quite naturally to questions about how optimistic or pessimistic people are about the current helping endeavor in general and particular aspects, such as the family therapy. One may wish to track changes in optimism and pessimism over time, in order to discern if there is a pattern of initial optimism followed by failure and pessimism and to discover if there has been any change at all. Some referrals are tainted with a tone of pessimism that remains throughout the work and generates a self-fulfilling prophecy, as when one is sent a "hopeless" case. During this discussion differences among the various helpers will also emerge. Such differences may be indicative of special relationships, frustrations between people, and fixed beliefs or prejudices.

Comparisons. Two categories of comparisons are often useful. In the first, family members may be asked to compare their experiences with the various helpers along a variety of dimensions. This may include comparisons of the kinds of help people have offered and what or whom family members have found the most helpful. Alliances and splits may emerge between family members and specific helpers. Themes of lack of differentiation of the various helpers by family members may also become apparent, as when the family indicate that they can see no differences among the helpers. It is important here to discern whether such lack of differentiation is because the helpers have simply made no impact collectively, whether the family is afraid to remark about differences for fear that the helpers might not like it, or whether the lack of permission to notice differences permeates the entire macrosystem (see the case below, "A Family Taking Care of Its Helpers").

Family members may also be asked to make comparisons between themselves and the helpers regarding who is more upset by what is presently occurring. During this portion of an interview one father remarked, much to the surprise of the assembled helpers, that he believed the helpers were far more upset and were indeed working harder than he was to solve the problem of his delinquent daughter.

A second major category of comparison is to ask the helpers to compare this family or specific members to other families with whom they have worked. Here the helpers' ideas about success and failure easily become available. Whether this family is a favorite with particular helpers also becomes clear, as do themes of sympathy, pity, dislike, frustration, and so on.

These questions regarding the present relationships in the macrosystem are by no means exhaustive. As one utilizes these suggested questions, other possibilities will appear, tailored to the specific situation of the macrosystem.

Future

Following this exploration, it is often useful to inquire about people's ideas of the future, including everyone's views of the family's future, the identified patient's future, and future relationships between the family and larger systems. It is during this section of the interview that previously unspoken plans that a particular helper may have will be raised. It is important that the consultant not get drawn into giving an opinion about such plans at this juncture but rather discusses what all of the participants think regarding the efficacy of such plans. One is frequently able to illuminate how such future plans may simply be "more of the same wrong solution" (Watzlawick, Weakland, & Fisch, 1974), replicating prior attempts. Further, one may be able to ask questions that lead to a discussion of how to make this new plan truly different by altering the interaction patterns that underpin its inception.

The consultant may wish to pose a variety of hypothetical scenarios to all assembled. It is often useful to juxtapose a future in which there is more help from more larger systems interacting with the family with a future in which outside help ceases, and to ask people what they believe would happen under these different sets of circumstances. The purpose of such questions is not to recommend either of these courses of action but to pose possibilities that are not presently available in the macrosystem. Family members' wishes for a nonexistent perfect helper may become clear in a macrosystem marked by the addition of more and more helpers. Analogic responses to a discussion of a future without help often indicate whether anyone envisions such a scenario as even remotely possible. Scenarios that suggest the exit of a particular helper often yield information about special alliances. Questions regarding for whom a future without helping efforts would be the hardest may reveal a belief that it would be harder for particular helpers than it would be for the family members (see the case below, "The More Help, the More Helplessness").

Participants' Questions

When the consultant has concluded his or her questions, it is beneficial to ask if the participants have any questions they wish to raise before a break. Sometimes people have come to the interview with particular issues they want to bring up, and they may consider the whole interview a waste of time if they do not have the opportunity to raise these. A helper may want tacit permission to leave a case and may take this opportunity to state this. Or a helper may wish to request greater contact among the professionals. A family member may choose to challenge a particular point of view. During this usually short portion of the interview, the consultant serves as a facilitator, taking note of the issues raised, for possible use in the intersession discussion.

At this point, the consultant must make a decision whether or not to ask all participants to wait, whether to conclude the interview in its entirety and send any ideas to the family therapist with instructions to send copies to all, or whether to ask the family and family therapist to wait for conclusions. Many times this decision is based on time constraints of the participants. If one or more of the helpers have to leave, it is best to thank and dismiss all of the helpers, except the family therapist who asked for the consultation. The family may or may not be asked to remain, depending on the plan for the intervention. Further, if it is discerned that the various helpers would resent being asked to wait while a team meets without them, then it is best to communicate the conclusions by mail to all of the helpers. The consultant makes his or her decision based on ideas about boundaries that have appeared during the interview. If one believes that a useful way to intervene may be to draw a boundary between the helpers and the family, then the end-of-session intervention may be given only to the family, as in the following case. (The specific intervention design will be described in Chapter 5.)

CASE EXAMPLE: A FAMILY TAKING CARE OF ITS HELPERS

A family therapist requested a family–larger system consultation. A family with whom he had been working appeared to be deteriorating over the last several weeks. At the same time, the therapist discovered that the family interacted regularly with many other helpers, some of whom were also expressing concern about the family.

The family consisted of a mother, Cathy Lee, 28, a father, Jim Lee, 29, and two children, Billy 4, and Christie, 2 (see Figure 4-1).

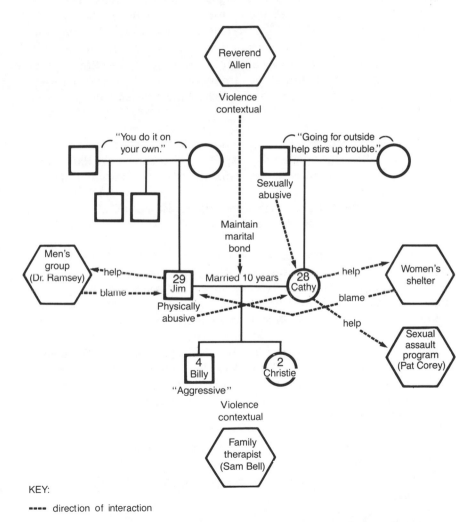

KEY:

---- direction of interaction

Figure 4-1. The Lee family genogram and conflicting perceptions and interactions.

The family originally came to family therapy presenting "aggressive behavior" in Billy. Over the course of 3 months in therapy, the family also told the therapist that Jim had beaten Cathy on many occasions. While the violence had ceased, both expressed fear that it could occur again. Shortly before the requested consultation, Cathy told the therapist that she had been sexually abused by her father when she was a child and young adolescent. The Lees had come to family therapy on the advice of their family physician, who knew only of the problems with Billy. On their own, they had also become involved with several other systems shortly before and shortly after commencing family therapy. The husband had joined a structured group for men who batter their wives. Cathy sought help for the prior incest, at a sexual assault program for women. Finally, the couple had become quite involved with the minister at their church and turned to him for counseling. By the time of the family–larger system interview, the family was regularly interacting with representatives of five larger systems. The larger systems involved included the following:

1. Women's Shelter—two counselors
2. Sexual assault program—paraprofessional counselor, Pat Corey
3. Local hospital forensic department, group for battering men—psychologist, Dr. Ramsey
4. Family therapy program—family therapist, Sam Bell
5. Church—minister, Reverend Allen

The family therapist set up the interview and invited the various participants. When he first discussed the possibility of such a meeting with the couple, they were very enthusiastic, informed the therapist of their close relationship to their minister, and requested that he also be invited. It is not unusual to discover more helpers than one knew about, in the process of setting up such an interview. When inviting the various helpers, the therapist also found that the two counselors at the Women's Shelter were the most alarmed about Cathy's recent behavior in group therapy, stating that she had become very distraught in recent sessions. At the same time they declined to come to the interview, stating that the group had just ended and they did not currently consider Cathy a client. Dr. Ramsey was reluctant to come, stating that he felt joint meetings were seldom useful, but he agreed to come. Reverend Allen and Pat Corey readily agreed to come.

During the family–larger system interview, several salient issues emerged.

1. The couple treated all of the helpers with great deference and politeness, refusing to draw any distinctions among them and insisting

that the best help resulted from a combination of people. The helpers treated each other with this same tone of politeness and initially minimized any differences among them. In fact, the differences in approaches and fundamental beliefs about the nature of the couple's problems were quite great. For instance, the structured group for battering men in which Jim was involved was a 5-year program, utilizing highly confrontational techniques and locating the cause of the violence in Jim, while the family therapy was based on a systemic model, was short term, and located the violence in the context of the couple's interaction. During the course of the interview, it emerged that Reverend Allen also saw the violence contextually, while Cathy felt that the counselors from the Women's Shelter certainly blamed Jim exclusively.

2. In response to questions regarding their view of the couple's marriage, all of the helpers except Reverend Allen stated that they believed they were neutral towards whether the couple stayed together or not. In fact, the various approaches and interventions utilized by the various helpers had a decidedly nonneutral effect on the couple's marriage. An implicit message from both the shelter and the men's group program was that this was not a good marriage and was perhaps not worth saving. The myth of neutrality added to the difficulty of drawing distinctions among the various helpers and their impact on the couple's relationship. Cathy and Jim stated that they were certainly not neutral and wanted to preserve their marriage.

3. During a portion of the interview devoted to the beliefs and attitudes of Jim's and Cathy's families towards outside help, it became clear that both came from families that did not believe in professional help. Jim said, "My father's view was 'you do it on your own,'" while Cathy said her family was adamantly against going for any outside help and told her she was a troublemaker for doing so. It also emerged that neither family of origin was particularly supportive to the couple. Cathy said, "My parents' view is, you made your bed—sleep in it!" An interesting pattern emerged, that when the couple visited either family of origin, they were unable to comment on any differences they observed, and they would end up fighting with each other.

4. During a discussion of what happened after each member of the couple had seen one of the helpers individually, a pattern emerged that they would discuss the session together, be unable to comment on differences among the helpers, and end up fighting with each other. This pattern appeared to be isomorphic with the pattern involving visits to their families of origin. In each situation, Cathy and Jim seemed unaware that the fights actually involved many people other than just the two of them and instead considered the fighting as further evidence that they were a bad couple. Fighting after sessions with the various helpers had become particularly bad in the last several weeks, when the input from the

various helpers had become particularly intense. The couple referred several times to this period as an "upheaval."

5. Any attempt by the consultant to connect the couple's current state of upheaval to the very different opinions they were hearing from the helpers was met with protection of the helpers by the couple. This theme of protection further emerged as it became apparent that the couple were very careful not to burden any one helper with their problems and that they carefully compartmentalized their troubles in order to avoid "blowing any of the helpers away." Jim reported that 3 years earlier they had tried going to one helper only and that they could tell that "it was hard on him" to hear all of their difficulties. In addition, the couple was very careful not to offend any of the helpers by pointing out differences among them. During this portion of the interview the various helpers appeared quite surprised.

6. During a discussion of future help, Cathy and Jim predicted a time when they would not need help but could not specify when this would be. At this juncture, three of the helpers began to talk of more help they could offer.

At the close of the interview, the consultant decided to have only the couple remain to hear the final intervention. One of the helpers had to leave, and it seemed better to draw a graphic boundary between the family and all of the helpers. As the interview drew to a close, the couple stood up, greeted all of the helpers warmly, hugged some of them, and thanked them profusely for taking their time to come to the interview.

The consultant and team met to discuss the session and plan an intervention. Utilizing several of the assessment concepts discussed in Chapter 3, the team saw many crucial areas. Competing definitions of the problem and approaches to solutions existed in the macrosystem. An escalating pattern regarding help existed: more and more help appeared to be required as more and more help was given. An unusual complementarity reversed the usual relation of clients and helpers, as the couple worked very hard to "take care" of the helpers. Triads were formed when the couple allied with various helpers and fought with each other regarding these alliances. Such triadic patterns appeared to replicate the couple's relationships with their families of origin.

The boundaries between Cathy and Jim seemed very diffuse, as did the boundaries between the couple and the various helpers. Until this session, the boundaries among the various helpers had been very rigid. Some did not even know of each other's existence, and no information had been exchanged regarding their various involvements with the couple. Several myths and beliefs permeated the macrosystem, some of which are important to reemphasize. The couple believed that they "had too many problems for one helper" and that it was their job to take care of the helpers. Dr. Ramsey and the Women's Shelter believed that there was only one way to deal with family violence and that the violence existed in Jim, while the family therapist and Reverend Allen believed that there were multiple ways to deal with the violence and that the violence was contextual. All of the helpers except Reverend Allen held the myth that they were neutral towards the ongoing existence of the couple's marriage. The solution behavior of all of the helpers, except the family therapist, and of the couple towards the issue of help was to favor specialization and more help. These various ideas led the team to develop an intervention that would potentially introduce clearer boundaries in the macrosystem and would utilize the unusual complementarity of a couple taking care of its helpers, by putting them "in charge" of their helpers. The intervention was designed to go with the system of specialization and compartmentalization, rather than challenge it. Finally, the intervention was intended to draw the couple together in a cooperative problem-solving venture and interrupt their fighting about help.

CONSULTANT: Let me tell you what we're thinking at this point, it's something we're hoping will be helpful to you in working with all of the people that you've got working with you. You have a big group of people, a fine group of people, engaged with you. However, what I think became apparent to me during the session is that the different input and, especially when it gets heavy, input from any one of the helpers, runs the risk of jamming up the two of you, and then you start fighting with each other, and you can't get clear as to what's causing what. That's not unusual in our experience, when there's a family and there's a lot of people trying to give them a hand, okay?

Now, one of the things I think you identified here this morning, and all of the helpers identified, is there are really distinct areas all of the helpers practice in, and which you agree are areas you need a hand in for the time being.

And that you find it more useful to have that kind of compartmentalized, which I think is fine. The problem is when it gets too heavy, and I think, from what I sensed from the two of you this morning, because you appreciate the help that people are extending to you, it may be a little hard to point out the differences between the helpers and say, "Halt, wait a minute, this is getting kind of overloaded for us," so you work very hard to try and keep peace between everybody and then the two of you end of fighting with each other. It's kind of like kids in a family sometimes when they don't want the parents to fight, so they don't point out any of the differences.

So let me give you a little tool that we just devised and suggest how we'd like you to use it. I'm going to draw it up on the board, then Sam's going to make one up for you, so you can take it home. So you don't need to worry about copying it down right now.

This is supposed to be a circle, a big circle. And let's divide it up into some parts here, kind of like a big pie, okay?

The idea is that each of these represents the various areas that the two of you are seeking and receiving some ideas in and some help in right now. So if we look, for instance, at the one area right here, the individual help for Jim regarding the issue of violence, right, and that that's primarily Dr. Ramsey's area—okay? [See Figure 4-2.]

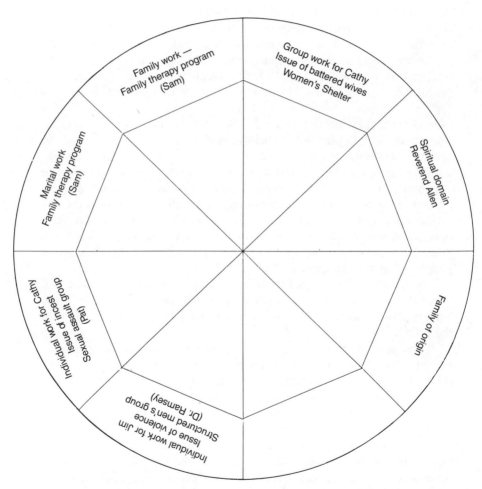

Figure 4-2. Tool used by the Lees to keep track of family–larger system interactions.

Note: The circle was drawn on a blackboard the size of an entire wall, metaphorically expressing the size of the issues of couple–helper interaction.

And then we might look and say there's individual work here for Cathy regarding the incest—and that that's primarily Pat and the sexual assault group—okay?

And then, that there's marital work for both of you and that that's primarily work with Sam and the family therapy program, and I think we'll draw a distinction here between marital and family work where the two of you would want to be looking at issues with your children, and that that's the work you also do primarily with Sam and the family therapy program. There's the work that Cathy's been involved in, that you've put on hold and you might reenter it or not reenter it, work regarding battered women, so that's Cathy and that's the work at the Women's Shelter—okay?

Then there's the whole spiritual domain, for you as a couple, and as a family and individually, and that's then the work with Reverend Allen.

Also, there's probably, whether you always realize it or not, ideas, influences, forces from your families of origin that are affecting how things work for the two of you and sometimes putting pressure on you, we'll make a category for that—okay? And then, we'll leave a blank here in case anybody else enters the sphere—okay?

What we suggest the two of you do with this, and we're going to make this up for the two of you to take home, okay, and it will be made up with each of these sections having some compartments within it, and we'll work it out that there's about 10 in each one. What we would like you to do is, every week, at a specified time, you two decide—every Sunday afternoon, or whatever you want—we'd like you to sit down with this, and we want you to decide "where is our work, my work or our work, on each of these areas?" That is to say, if we think of this as number one and here as number 10, number one being the least heavy, least intense, mild, soft, and over here, things getting really heavy and intense, upheaval—okay? So that you get a chart every week so that you start to see, if you visualize where I am going here with this, *you would know* when it's getting to be too much in more than one area, and that one area at a time is probably all anyone can really manage in terms of really looking at heavy, heavy stuff. [See Figure 4-3.]

And any time any two areas go over say five, when you start to fill this in, that's a warning signal, and I think the two of you could use a warning signal together and then if it starts to move to more than two of these, three or four of these and they are into the sevens and eights, whoa, it is time to say we really need to make some new decisions here, about where do we really want to focus for the next 2 months, like this—do you follow my meaning? (Couple nod yes.)

So this is something that'll really be a resource to the two of you, and we're going to give you several copies of it today, and when you run out, you can take the last one and you can make some more copies of it, so

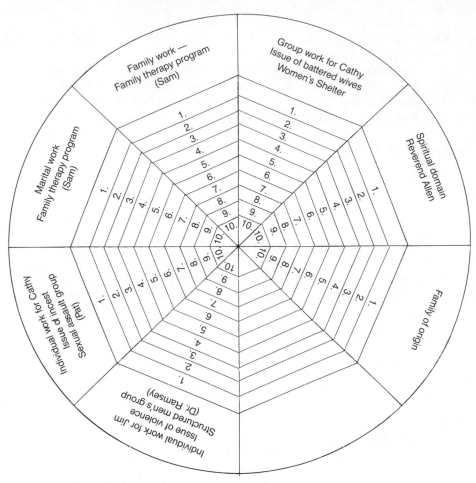

Figure 4-3. Tool for Lees' problems with numbers signifying increasing intensity.

that you'll have that, and then when you need to, *you'll* be able to let the helpers know, "Wait a minute, it's time for us to cool out a little bit, because we're recognizing we've got three 7's," and that together, that the two of you decide which one do we want to move on for the time being—okay?

Sam's going to send a copy of this to all of the people that were here this morning, so that it won't seem kind of crazy to them that this is going on and *you will be in charge of how much help you need, when you need it, and whom you need it from.*

The couple came back in a month to see the family therapist. They began by describing how they had used the instrument that had been given to them at the consultation. Rather than doing it together, each had done it privately, and they discussed it together later. This interesting variation on the instructions was, in fact, the first time the couple had not exactly followed what a helper had asked them to do. It also appeared to enhance clearer boundaries between them and to allow for the peaceful exchange of different points of view. They said they felt closer and more positive towards each other than they had for a long time. They had seen no helpers during the month, except Reverend Allen. They were going out as a couple, which they had not done for several years. They had joined a church group with other couples and were beginning to make friends. Cathy stated, "Maybe if we had more friends, we'd need fewer helpers!" Their son had been much less aggressive, and they felt they were being firmer with him. They dropped plans they had been making to put him in a group for "aggressive boys" at the Women's Shelter. Finally, they said they had visited each of their families of origin at Christmas after a long separation. Prior to the visits they agreed to support each other and not turn on each other as they always had done previously, and they succeeded in this.

Following the family–larger system interview, the family therapist and the counselor from the sexual assault program agreed to be in touch in order to make sure that each one's work was not interfering with the other's. The psychologist declined to be involved, stating that Jim was really in a follow-up phase of the 5-year program, during which he would only be contacted once every 6 months.

Family therapy was terminated by mutual agreement 3 months after the consultation. At the 1-year follow-up the couple reported doing very well. Violence had not reoccurred. Their only involvement with an outside system (other than work and school) was their church, which they continued to find satisfying. The wife also reported feeling much more freedom to do things independently, without her husband feeling threatened. Finally, she stated that she had confronted her father regarding his sexual abuse of her. She was not seeing helpers at the time and said she simply decided the time had come to do so. Her confidence in her capacity to initiate and handle this conversation had not been seen earlier.

The family–larger system interview in this case had several important effects. Like many such interviews, it was an intervention per se among the helpers. Prior to this interview, they had never met and were not fully cognizant of each other's existence. The interview, which highlighted differences among the helpers and the impact of these differences on the couple's interactions, gave the helpers and the couple a new way to conceptualize current difficulties. The questions and responses wove a theme in which the couple's problems could be located not only at an individual or couple level but also at a macrosystemic level. Information generated in the interview was then utilized to design an intervention that focused on couple–helper complementarity and couple–helper boundaries.

In the following consultation the interview clarified the intricate pattern of interaction among the family and their helpers. The helpers' conflicting advice was used as the foundation for an intervention promoting the parent's empowerment and autonomy.

CASE EXAMPLE: THE MORE HELP, THE MORE HELPLESSNESS

A consultation was requested by a family therapist for a case involving recurring school refusal by a 15-year-old boy. The therapist requested the consultation for two reasons. The case had an erratic history of slight progress followed by relapse followed by slight progress, and so on. The school guidance counselor had called the therapist several times, urgently requesting that "more be done," while the therapist was following a course of backing off. Thus a treatment triangle existed (see Figure 4-4).

The family consisted of a mother, Mrs. Clark, age 39, the identified patient Ron, age 15, and a daughter, Karen, age 13. The parents had been divorced 12 years. The father left following the birth of Karen, who was developmentally disabled. No one in the family had heard from him for 11 years. Mrs. Clark described him as "irresponsible and alcoholic." Mrs. Clark also came from a single-parent family and described her father as "irresponsible and alcoholic." Ron had been an excellent student until reaching adolescence, when he became severely depressed and refused to go to school.

Present at the consulting interview were the three members of the nuclear family, the family therapist, and the school guidance counselor. The interview began with a discussion of the various efforts tried in the previous 15 months. The intent of this line of questioning was to discover the range of the family's involvements with helpers, their beliefs and attitudes towards help, how the helpers saw the efforts tried, and so on.

CONSULTANT: What have you tried in an effort to solve this?

MOTHER: Well, when he first got depressed, I took him to see Dr. Peter Cook, a psychiatrist, Bob here (*pointing to guidance counselor*) thought I should do that.

CONSULTANT: What did Dr. Cook suggest?

MOTHER: He put him in the hospital. He was there a month.

CONSULTANT: Did that make the situation better or worse?

MOTHER: It improved for a little while, and then it got worse.

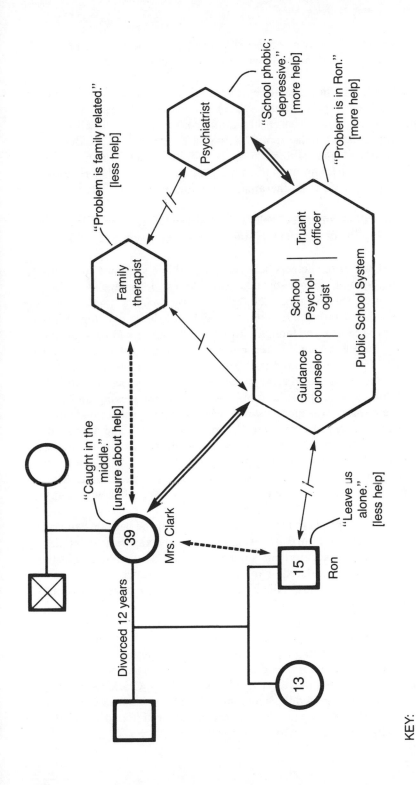

KEY:
═══ alliance
─/─ conflict
▪▪▪▪ problematic link

Figure 4-4. The Clark family and outside systems: Triangulation due to conflicting problem definitions.

"Problem is family related." [less help]

"School phobic; depressive." [more help]

"Problem is in Ron." [more help]

Psychiatrist

Family therapist

Truant officer

School Psychol- ogist

Guidance counselor

Public School System

"Caught in the middle." [unsure about help]

Mrs. Clark

Divorced 12 years

39

15

Ron

"Leave us alone." [less help]

13

127

This was the first of many examples that the family and the two professionals relate of slight improvement followed by a relapse of greater severity.

All the helpers who had entered the Clark family sphere were male. They included a school counselor whose ostensible job was to counsel Ron but who saw Mrs. Clark in her home once a week and called her daily; a psychiatrist who placed both Ron and Mrs. Clark on antidepressant medication; a truant officer who arrived daily to take Ron to school; a school psychologist who insisted that Ron had a phobia that required hospitalization; and a family therapist who counseled vigorously against hospitalization.

In a consulting interview held with the family and the helpers in order to sort out the tangle and facilitate a course of action, the following emerged.

The majority of the helpers believed the problem stemmed from this being a single-parent, female-headed family with a teenage boy. The mother accepted this, stating that "it's because we're a single-parent family. If he had a father all along, this wouldn't be happening. We'd have had more input in the family, and I wouldn't have had to go so far outside the family for help." Karen concurred, stating that "he needs a Big Brother." Ron also believed that his mother was unable to function on her own, and managed to arrange for several male helpers to interact with her. Thus, a belief that the family was somehow lacking and that normal development was not possible was held by professionals and family members. Strengths in the mother remained hidden and untapped.

Mrs. Clark and the guidance counselor were on a first-name basis. He called her frequently and stopped by the house. While evidently concerned about Ron, he was presently more concerned about Mrs. Clark's well-being. He was usually the initiator of each new helping attempt.

Mrs. Clark felt pressured to accept the advice of the various helpers, who treated her with a mixture of kindness and exasperation at her seeming inability to execute their suggestions, due to Ron's refusal to cooperate. The helpers offered or insisted on a wide range of strategies, dragging Ron to school, hospitalizing Ron, leaving Ron alone to sort out his own difficulties, medicating Ron, and so on, all requiring Mrs. Clark to be responsible for implementing their suggestions within a context that had designated her as incomplete, helpless, and enmeshed with her son. In response to a line of inquiry regarding the hypothetical cessation of help, Ron said, "My mother would be hurting less. She feels she needs to get help, but all it does is make her feel helpless!" Mrs. Clark responded, "Well, I'd be out of the middle. The way it's gone is whoever is at that point helping us is on our side, Ron is on the other side and me in the middle; so whatever I do is wrong with somebody!"

At the time of the consulting interview with the helpers and the family, the helpers were in conflict with one another regarding the correct diagnosis and course of action. Each believed it was his place to steer the family in a particular direction (e.g., hospitalization, truancy approaches, backing off), and none approached Mrs. Clark as a person capable of making her own decisions, once given a range of information and options.

The consultant explored what people believed would happen if all help were to stop, suggesting that at 15 or 16 many youngsters decide to quit school. This was balanced with a line of questions exploring the next intervention being suggested by the guidance counselor, namely hospitalization at the local Children's Hospital, a setting not previously tried. The consultant remained neutral towards both possibilities and utilized the questions to draw a distinction between no help and more help and between normalcy and psychiatric patient. As might be expected, the two helpers split, with the guidance counselor favoring hospitalization and predicting a terrible future if all help ceased and the family therapist favoring less help. Ron believed he would do well in a few years "if everyone got off my back so I could think!" Karen preferred Ron to go to the hospital and "stop bugging" her. Most interesting was Mrs. Clark's response, "If all help stopped, I think he would pull himself together in about 10 years. In fact, my brother quit school at 15, and now he's an engineer. So for a while, he'd probably be a bum, but he'd get on his feet." Regarding the hospital, Mrs. Clark stated (looking at the guidance counselor), "Ron would hate me if I make him go, but it might just be the best thing." Clearly, the mother was caught between supporting her son and supporting the guidance counselor, who was the primary adult male in her life. As a result, her messages to her son were duplicitous, and Ron responded with increased confusion, thereby supporting the view that he was a patient. The periods of brief improvement followed by relapse were both a metaphor for the family's relationship to helpers and a way to ensure that helpers remain in the family sphere.

Questions answered during the interview by the family and helpers indicated several problem areas suggested by the family–larger system assessment model. An escalating pattern of complementarity permeated the macrosystem. As more and more helpers offered services to Mrs. Clark, she became more and more helpless. In turn, as she attempted to carry out the helpers' advice with her son, he appeared more and more helpless.

Conflicts among the helpers, especially the guidance counselor and the family therapist, served to triangulate Mrs. Clark, who felt pressed to agree with each but, of course, could not do so.

Myths about single parents and about mothers and sons were rampant in the macrosystem, as all agreed that single parents were limited, single-parent families were flawed, and sons in such families needed male role models, rather than strong, decisive mothers.

Mrs. Clark was in a particular bind, as she was being urged to depend on helpers, while being subtly criticized for her "helplessness."

All of these assessment ideas, generated from the interview, were utilized to develop an intervention. The consultant designed an intervention with the deliberate intent of restoring the decision-making role to Mrs. Clark, as head of her family. In view of the conflicting advice on hospitalizing Ron, the consultant suggested an experiment to Mrs. Clark.

CONSULTANT: You have let us know today that the most difficult issue you face at the present is whether to hospitalize Ron or not hospitalize Ron. Or perhaps another way of putting it, is whether to hospitalize Ron or back off of any treatment and go with Ron's idea that if people got off his back, he'd be able to work things out. I would like to suggest an experiment for you to do, designed, we hope, to produce greater clarity and help you reach a decision, because ultimately you're in charge. We suggest you divide the week in the following way: On Saturday, Monday, and Wednesday, we want you to adopt the position that Ron is going to the hospital. On those days, you should research everything you need to regarding hospitalization. You can talk to doctors, you can talk to other mothers who have hospitalized their children, you can talk to people who have been to the hospital, you can talk to the guidance counselor about it and to your mother. On those days, we want you to regard Ron as a patient, since that's what he will be, and we want you to talk to him with conviction about why you think it's a good idea for him to go to the hospital. You should do this regardless of how Ron responds.

Then, on Sunday, Tuesday, and Thursday, we want you to adopt the position that Ron is a normal boy who has decided to quit school for a while and, therefore, no helping efforts are necessary. On those days, you should take note of all the ways Ron is just a regular boy. You should review on those days all of the failures, all of the previous advice from the various men who have tried to give you a hand with this. If anyone calls you on those days to talk about help for Ron or to give you advice, we suggest you say, "I think we should leave him alone." On those days, you would talk to Ron with conviction about why no help is needed, and that he's a normal boy. Then take Friday off and start again. We'd like you to do this for about 3 weeks or until you feel the issues have been clarified.

Immediately after this experiment was described, the guidance counselor solicited Ron's opinion, rather than Mrs. Clark's. Ron challenged his mother to reengage in a familiar struggle that often left her feeling helpless: "I'm just telling you—if you send me to the hospital, you'll never see me again!"

In earlier similar challenges, Mrs. Clark had anxiously turned to one of the helpers, who immediately intervened, told her what to do, and became parental toward both Ron and her. On this day, she simply got up, put on her coat, and said to Ron, "Well, that's something we'll have to discuss if and when that happens. Today is a Friday. Today is a 'nothing' day. I'm not going to discuss it!"

After carrying out this experiment, Mrs. Clark decided not to hospitalize Ron and to limit her involvement with professional helpers to one for her own issues. It is interesting to note that she chose a woman counselor. This outcome exemplifies ways in which a macrosystemic perspective can effectively feed back on individual developmental needs, previously invisible due to macrosystemic patterns and constraints. Ron returned to school and completed his spring examinations with success. Since Ron was now attending school and Mrs. Clark was pursuing her own therapy, the interest of helpers in the family dissipated.

The consultant in this case focused on eliciting and interdicting the patterns between the various helpers and Mrs. Clark that, in fact, were exacerbating her sense of helplessness and confusion. The interview also focused on Mrs. Clark's strengths and affirmed this single-parent family as whole and complete. The intervention, rather than giving Mrs. Clark more advice, shifted her position vis-à-vis helpers and highlighted her ability to make decisions for herself and her family.

EFFECTS OF THE INTERVIEW ON THE FAMILY–LARGER SYSTEM RELATIONSHIPS

The family–larger system interview is an intervention in the family–helpers relationship, even when no formal end-of-session intervention is utilized. Often, just the preparation for the interview begins to evoke changes in the macrosystem, as some helpers may begin to distance or draw firmer boundaries, while the existence of hitherto unknown helpers may be discovered.

The coming together of family members and helpers at a meeting in which all are interviewed is a very unusual event. Helpers are used to meeting in the clients' absence to discuss them, while families are used to being the only ones who are interviewed. The sheer unexpectedness of the family–larger system interview may facilitate the thawing of frozen relationships. Gathering together for such an interview is often an intervention in boundaries, as people who are crucially involved in a situation may be meeting each other for the first time. This pertains both to multiple helpers who are involved with a family and may have never spoken, much less discovered that their work may be at cross purposes, and family members who may have never met or spoken with helpers who are involved with individual members and may be having a powerful impact on family relationships, as in the case of the Lees discussed above.

The interview, especially in its initial stages, is often an enactment of all of the existing relationships in a highly condensed manner and thus has the potential for being a graphic, paradoxical prescription of the entire macrosystem. Occasionally elements of absurdity are highlighted, as when three family members and 15 helpers assemble for a meeting.

As the interview unfolds through the consultant's careful and respectful questioning, participants begin to make discoveries about their relationships. For instance, following a family–larger system interview, a probation officer remarked, "I found out that I'm working harder than the family is to get things changed, and I think my working harder may well be contributing to their working less hard! I think I'm going to relax a bit and see what happens." Such discoveries may facilitate the development of new relationships in the macrosystem and new directions for the family and for individual members.

CHAPTER 5

Intervention Design and Implementation

Designing interventions for the family–larger system configuration is a more complex and difficult task than designing interventions intended solely for the family context. While many aspects of intervention design that are familiar to family therapists may be utilized, one must also attend to aspects that are particular to macrosystemic work. As described in Chapter 4, the family–larger system interview is an intervention per se. In the present chapter, attention is focused on end-of-session and post-session interventions.

Family–larger system interventions are designed to affect a more inclusive level than individual or family interventions. Even if the intervention is given to the family or one member of the family, the intention is to target the macrosystemic organization. In the interventions described in the two cases in Chapter 4, intervention directions were given to family members, but the effect was macrosystemic. Likewise, one may choose to intervene with a member of the larger system in a way that affects family–larger system relationships. Decisions regarding to whom to give a specific intervention may hinge on availability and clinical judgments regarding issues of cooperation, motivation, apparent hostility, symmetry, and so on.

In designing interventions to target the macrosystem, one is particularly interested in discovering isomorphic patterns and themes that repeat in varying forms at different levels. Interventions designed to affect the macrosystem may then be directed at such a pattern at one level and have a reverberating effect throughout the macrosystem. Recognition of such isomorphism can lead the consultant to design an intervention that is efficacious within the family, between the family and larger systems, and within the larger systems.

BRIEF EXAMPLE: AN INTERVENTION IN ISOMORPHIC PATTERNS

A family therapist requested a family–larger system interview. The family consisted of Mrs. Ward, 65, Mr. Ward, 75, and the identified patient

John, 28. The family had been involved with outsiders since John began having school problems at age 6 and was diagnosed "mentally retarded", a diagnosis that the family and helpers variously believed and disbelieved. The ambiguity of this diagnosis seemed to underpin a lack of definiteness in everyone's behavior vis-à-vis John. Presently, John refused to go to work or help around the house. He drank and got into trouble with the law. He left home once and failed. Outsiders at the interview included John's probation officer, income security worker, and individual therapist, and the family therapist.

Isomorphism emerged in two ways during the interview. To begin, the family members were overprotective towards and exasperated with John. John responded to their overprotection with dangerous ploys and to their exasperation by an apologetic and endearing stance, thus continuing the cycle in a well-rehearsed range. In turn, the outside systems were overprotective towards and exasperated with the family. Helpers devoted extra hours to this case and had many case conferences to design plans for John and his family. Each plan was met with nodding agreement and enthusiasm by the family, just as the parents' plans for John were initially received by him. The parents would then ignore the plans of the outside systems, and John would ignore the plans of the parents. Periods of intense frustration and anger were followed by periods of humility and apology.

Secondly, within the family there was covert competition between the parents for who would eventually succeed with John. This covert competition was mirrored in a subtle symmetrical struggle among the outside systems for which one would come up with the appropriate "answers" for John. Finally, this same struggle was evident between the family and all of the larger systems, about who, in the final analysis, "knew best."

The consultant's intervention positively reframed and prescribed the isomorphic patterns, suggesting that John, although 28 years old, was developmentally more like 18 and needed his parents to tell him what to do, just as they needed him not to listen in order for him to individuate and for parents and son to separate. Similarly the outside systems, having been engaged for so long with this family and facing a difficult disengagement on both sides, needed to continue to develop plans, in order to help the family discover its own solutions, since the more plans the outsiders came up with the more the family went its own way, a difficult developmental task. Thus "help" in this case was reframed as most helpful when it appeared least helpful.

Following the delivery of this opinion, the parents stopped offering new plans to John, and the helpers stopped offering new plans to the parents. John's probation officer began to hold him more consistently accountable for his behavior, and the parents did likewise. John responded by attending and completing a job-training program and getting off probation. Cooperation in John's behalf, rather than competition, began to mark the macrosystem.

In focusing on isomorphic patterns and themes one is seeking to take particular care not to design interventions that replicate what already exists in the system. In the brief example above, the consultant's opinion was offered more as a tentative hunch than as an expert opinion, in order to avoid adding to the competitive struggle over who knew best. As well, the consultant took care not to offer any new plans for John, his family, or the helpers, since to do so would have been to replicate existing patterns.

Interventions in the family–larger system network should be presented with language and tone that communicates a sense of appreciation to the various participants in the macrosystem. Contributions that have worked should be selected out and confirmed. It is tempting, when larger systems are criticizing a family, to criticize the larger system in turn. Most often, however, this simply adds rigidity and no new information to the system. The use of affirmation to both family members and helpers often casts a new light on preexisting relationships. This is especially true when helpers have highlighted only deficits in the family, and family members have seen only negative aspects of the helpers. Further, affirmation by the consultant in the delivery of interventions is often unexpected by the participants in the family–larger system context, who frequently expect to hear criticism. This very quality of unexpectedness can begin to alter relationships, reduce suspicions, and open more productive negotiations among the participants.

Certain family–larger system interventions can be utilized in one context or setting, but not in another. One is looking at the dimension of permission to intervene. A session and subsequent intervention in a family therapy program may allow for very different possibilities than a session held at a public school or a residential facility.

BRIEF EXAMPLE: FAILURE TO APPRECIATE THE CONTEXT

A family consisting of a single-parent, recently widowed mother and her 15-year-old daughter was referred to a therapy project within a public school because the girl was refusing to attend school. Since the death of her father, the girl remained at home every day with her mother. The family came for sessions, but the girl continued to remain at home. Gradually, more and more school professionals became involved with the case, including two teachers, a guidance counselor, the principal, and the family therapy team from within the school. A consultation was arranged by the family therapy team, who requested that all involved attend. Many aspects of the macrosystemic organization emerged during the consultation, including a high level of conflict among school personnel regarding the best course of action, triadic relationships involving the family and school, and behavior on everyone's part that, in fact, supported the girl's staying home, including special arrangements, tutors, and daily visits by the counselor to the mother. After gathering this information, the consultant offered an opinion that positively connoted everyone's actions and prescribed no change, within a frame of reference that highlighted the girl's protection of her mother and the school's protection of the family during this time of grief. While the intervention made adequate sense out of the information generated at the interview, it was too out of sync with the school's sense of its mission, that is, to educate children. The school personnel became extremely angry, criticized the family therapy team for bringing in the consultant, and began to use punitive measures against the family. The consultant had failed to appreciate the school context and its unspoken norms and rules. While any effective intervention certainly must challenge existing constraints, it must do so in a way that is not so dissonant as to be dismissed out of hand or to lead to a worsening of the situation.

In designing any family–larger system intervention, one may ask the following questions:

1. Does the intervention target the macrosystem, regardless of the specific person or subsystem to whom the intervention is given?
2. Does the intervention utilize isomorphic patterns and themes in effective ways?
3. Does the intervention avoid replicating rigid patterns?
4. Does the intervention utilize affirmation, highlight preexisting resources, and make use of the unexpected?
5. Is the intervention designed and given with an appreciation of the context?

INTERVENTIONS TO DELINEATE AND REDISTRIBUTE TASKS

The simplest and most direct form of intervention with families and larger systems is that which delineates and/or redistributes tasks among the larger system representatives. Such an intervention generally arises out of a family–larger system session when it becomes apparent that family members and/or helpers have some confusion regarding whose job it is to do what task, *and* there is a fair to high degree of cooperation evident in the macrosystem. Often such sorting out of jobs and clarification of roles and boundaries will occur spontaneously during the interview, and remarks may be offered by the consultant at the end of the session to reaffirm such discoveries and agreements. For instance, in response to a line of questioning about to whom one could turn for particular issues, a family member may indicate that the family always turns to the school guidance counselor, even for matters outside of his appropriate sphere, or that the father confers only with his individual therapist, bypassing both the family and family therapist. As these discoveries emerge in the interview, often the helpers will begin to say, "That's not my job."

Sometimes a family's seeming inability to distinguish differences amongst helpers is an indication of a similar pattern among family members. Families with rules against noticing or commenting on differences among members will often be unable to comment on differences among helpers. In addition, if lines are sharply drawn in a family regarding side-taking and alliances, the family may distinguish helpers in this same "you're either for us or against us" mode and be unable to draw further distinctions among the helpers. If the helpers get inducted into this pattern, their work with the family will become confused and lack clarity regarding whose job is what.

BRIEF EXAMPLE: A FAMILY ADOPTS ITS HELPERS

A family consisting of a single mother and her three daughters was referred to family therapy by a local welfare department. The mother and her ex-husband had been imprisoned on felony charges for 10 years. During this time, the daughters, now 17, 16, and 14, were raised by the paternal grandparents. One year before the consultation, the mother had been released from prison and had regained custody of her daughters. The family was assigned a child-welfare worker, Ms. Grey, at that time. The mother and Ms. Grey formed a very close relationship. Soon the paternal grandparents began a custody suit for the three girls. Due both to the stress of the suit and the need to reconstitute the family, Ms. Grey sent the family for family therapy. Child welfare paid for the therapy. Conflict between the mother and the paternal grandparents escalated. As conflict escalated, several things began to happen. The family therapist, Ms. Williams, tried unsuccessfully to engage the grandparents in the therapy. The grandparents sent very critical letters about the mother to the therapist. The therapist, the welfare worker, and the mother grew closer. The daughters made the following moves: the eldest returned to the grandparents, the middle daughter moved in with friends, and the youngest remained with her mother and grew closer to her. The family therapist began to feel that her work was not going anywhere. She reported feeling stuck and asked for a consultation.

The mother, the youngest daughter, the welfare worker, and the family therapist came to the consultation. All others refused to attend. In response to questions regarding the welfare worker's interest in the family, Ms. Grey indicated that there were no abuse or neglect issues and that, in fact, she had no legitimate reason for keeping the case open. She stated that since the youngest child had recently begun to have some school problems, she could stay involved. The emergence of school problems seemed to coincide with some threat that Ms. Grey might need to stop interacting with the family.

The consultant asked the mother who she would call or turn to in times of need. She responded, "I call either Ms. Grey or Ms. Williams. I try one, and if I can't get her, then I try the other. It doesn't matter who I reach as long as I reach one of them." She drew no distinctions between the two helpers—they were simply on her side.

The consultant then asked the daughter "who was in the family currently," attempting to understand how she saw her sisters' positions. The answer was quite surprising, as she stated, "My family is me, my mother, Ms. Grey, and Ms. Williams. They are our aunties—they are sisters to my mother." The family members further elaborated that they experienced the helpers as on the family's side in a war with the paternal grandparents. Thus the helpers had fully joined a system in which there appeared to be only three positions, "with us" (like the mother and the youngest daughter), "against us" (on the grandparents' side, where the eldest daughter was now positioned), or "out" (where the middle daughter was). The position of being loyal to both sides, being able to work with or have contact with both sides, was presently nonexistent. The helpers' work was severely handicapped by this configuration.

The end-of-session intervention by the consultant was simply to draw a distinction between the work of the family therapist and the work of the welfare worker. This was done first by removing family therapy from the umbrella of welfare services for the family and reconstituting it as that which the family would negotiate for on their own. The family would pay a minimal amount for sessions, and reports would not be issued to the welfare department by the family therapist. The family therapist was then advised to adopt a coaching position with the mother in order to deal with extended family issues. The therapist had said during the session that she had been reluctant to do this earlier and had fallen into a position of supporting the mother, the same position as the welfare worker and the youngest daughter.

This intervention had the effect of more clearly delineating the roles of family therapist and welfare worker, freeing the family therapist from a stuck position, and allowing for the introduction of difference in the subsystem of mother and youngest daughter, ultimately allowing a fourth available position to emerge for the daughters, that of being loyal to both sides of the family.

Occasionally the consultant may wish to suggest an unusual redistribution of tasks in order to ultimately accomplish a clarification of roles and boundaries.

BRIEF EXAMPLE: FORMING A LIMITED PARTNERSHIP

A single-parent family consisting of a widowed mother, Mrs. Walton, and two adolescent children, Keith, 15, and Ann, 13, was sent to family therapy by Keith's probation officer, Ms. Green. She had been involved with Keith and the family for 2 years, during which time Mr. Walton had committed suicide. Immediately following the suicide, Ms. Green had extended her services far beyond the usual probation relationship and had become like a counselor to the whole family. Ultimately feeling overextended, she referred the family to family therapy. Unfortunately, the referral had not been explained very well, as Ms. Green told the family simply that her supervisor believed this would be best. She continued to see Keith weekly. The family went to family therapy very reluctantly. They liked Ms. Green very much and felt they had to go or that she might get into trouble with her supervisor. Rather than engage with the family therapist, however, the family was mostly silent at sessions. Family issues continued to be worked out by Keith's discussing them with Ms. Green and returning to his family with whatever Ms. Green had said. This set of issues emerged at a family–larger system interview, along with the information that the family felt it would be disloyal to Ms. Green if they were to engage with the family therapist. Ms. Green also stated that Keith kept asking her to see his mother and sister and that she kept referring him back to the family therapist. There was a high degree of respect and good will between the probation officer and the family therapist. She had referred other cases to him that had gone very well, indicating that the present circumstances were unusual. For these reasons the consultant decided to suggest a redistribution of roles that did not follow the usual job descriptions but would lead to a clarification of roles and boundaries. Following the session, the consultant sent this memo to the family therapist, with copies to Ms. Green and the family. (Memos as interventions will be discussed below.)

> Thank you for the opportunity to conduct a consultation with you regarding Keith Walton, his family, and Keith's probation officer, Ms. Green.
> It would seem that Ms. Green's referral of the family to this program was quite appropriate, and that she was sensitive in recognizing this need. What appears to be the case, however, is that your work with the family has been missing significant input, which I feel you would most successfully gain through Ms. Green's help, as she provided in this meeting.
> I recognize that what I would be suggesting, in requesting Ms. Green's help, would be a difficult thing, in that she stated that her goal is to get the

family on its own feet so that Keith no longer misbehaves in ways that require her involvement. It appears to me, though, that perhaps this needs to be a gradual process. I would recommend your using her knowledge and connection with the family as an asset to the therapy that you do. I would suggest that between now and May, when the court will be reviewing Keith's probation, you request that Ms. Green attend your meetings with the family and meet with you just prior to each session to help you be brought up to date.

I believe that your forming a partnership with Ms. Green in this way would be useful in avoiding confusion and making sure that the family is not given conflicting advice and suggestions. Particularly, given that the same issues are being discussed with the family by you and Ms. Green, it would seem most effective to combine your respective resources.

I would suggest that this arrangement might be reviewed in May, following Keith's court appearance.

In the meantime, perhaps you can contact Ms. Green to arrange a time that will be mutually convenient for her and the family to schedule a next appointment.

The effect of this suggestion, which at first may sound like it increases Ms. Green's involvement with the family, was, in fact, to attenuate it. She stopped her weekly meetings with Keith, replacing these with meetings every 2 or 3 weeks with the family and the family therapist. She was able to utilize the family's affection for her to effect a positive engagement with the family therapist. After three sessions, her presence at family therapy sessions was no longer needed. Keith got off probation, and the family concluded a successful therapy.

The suggested redistribution of roles in unusual ways should only be utilized when one has a clear and complete sense of the larger system's mandates and requirements. In the case just discussed, the consultant knew that the probation officer would be able to form a limited partnership, see Keith less often, and still fulfill her mandate as a probation officer. The consultant knew further that the family therapist would welcome this arrangement and would not feel undercut. Finally, it was clear from the interview that the family was already telling Ms. Green all manner of family issues, such that boundaries were not made more diffuse by the intervention, but were ultimately made clearer.

Ritual Interventions

Ritual interventions are among the most creative and useful in systemic family therapy. Rituals designed to intervene in family patterns have been described by many practitioners (Imber-Black, 1986a, 1986b, 1988;

Imber Coppersmith, 1985c; Mandanes, 1981; Selvini Palazzoli *et al.*, 1978b; Papp, 1980). Rituals differ from tasks most notably in that rituals are designed to allow for greater spontaneity and inventiveness on the part of the participants. Rituals frequently involve symbols and symbolic actions, capable of multiple meanings. Thus, while tasks tend to target only behavior, rituals target behavior, cognition, and affect.

Sociocultural and therapeutic rituals share several functions. Rituals may reduce anxiety about change. Since rituals often utilize that which is familiar, in a time-bounded and space-bounded manner, change is experienced as manageable by the participants. Ritual promotes action and new ways of doing, that which in turn may alter thoughts and beliefs and relationship options. Since rituals may alter social structure and facilitate the coordination of individual, family, larger system, and community levels, they are useful for altering the family–larger system relationship.

Rituals designed for families and larger systems are often unusual and unexpected and may, therefore, facilitate the generation of new patterns and possibilities in formerly rigid macrosystems.

Transition Rituals

For families, transition rituals are designed and utlized to mark developmental transitions. Families may have normative transition rituals (e.g., weddings, baptisms, bar mitzvahs, funerals), or therapeutic rituals may be designed to mark and facilitate transitions. Often transition rituals highlight both internal family and individual member changes *and* changes in the family's relationship to the wider community. Thus transition rituals are a useful category of intervention to mark and facilitate changes in the macrosystem, targeting the family, the larger systems, and their relationship to each other.

Engagement Rituals

For some families, the transition from being a family that is extremely isolated, with no outside input, to becoming a family that can effectively engage with larger systems is a difficult transition. Such families are often sent for help by others, particularly by physicians or school personnel who may interact with one member and discern a need for family intervention. At times, such referrals are not adequately explained to the family, who feel blamed or intimidated. It is not unusual for such families to come for help to a therapist or counselor, but be quite confused regarding what to expect and what it is safe to discuss. Rather than considering the family uncooperative, the larger system representative may wish to consider an engagement ritual designed to assist the family from an isolated position to a connected position.

BRIEF EXAMPLE: THE PROS AND CONS OF DISCUSSING SENSITIVE
ISSUES OPENLY

A family consisting of two parents and two children, Bruce, 8, and an infant daughter, had been referred for family therapy by Bruce's school because of what was labeled "babyish" behavior at school, recently including eneuresis. The boy had refused to talk to the school psychologist, who then came to believe that there must be secrets in the family. The family arrived for family therapy under duress from larger systems. During the interview, two salient pieces of information emerged: the family had never talked to outsiders about anything, and they regarded the referral as blameful and punitive. Both parents came from families where "you did not take your problems to outsiders." While they were alarmed about Bruce's behavior, they felt constrained from discussing their concerns with anyone outside the family and had begun to discuss it less at home since the school began to pressure them to go to therapy. During the session, the parents showed great concern about talking in front of Bruce and asked that he leave the room.

A ritual was designed to target the family's relationship to outsiders and put any decisions about changing the rule about talking with outsiders in the family's hands. The parents were told that therapy generally involved "discussing sensitive issues openly," that very often such discussion was beneficial for families, but that only they knew what would be best for their family. Thus, the therapist positioned herself as less expert than the family on the issues of the family's relationship to outsiders. Since the family's relationship to the school had been one where they felt put down, the therapist's stance was quite unexpected. The therapist then suggested to the family that they have the following talks:

1. The mother and father were to discuss the pros and cons of discussing sensitive issues openly in their family and with an outsider.
2. The mother and Bruce were to discuss the pros and cons of discussing sensitive issues openly in their family and with an outsider.
3. The father and Bruce were to discuss the pros and cons of discussing sensitive issues openly in their family and with an outsider.
4. The mother and father were to meet again to discuss all of the other discussions.

The family was asked to call the therapist when they were ready. The family called in 2 weeks and asked for an appointment. They came in together and were eager to talk about what had happened. During the father's discussion with Bruce, the boy began to tell him what was troubling him at home and at school. Bruce had never before spoken to his father about his concerns, which included the father's recent unemployment, the mother's going to work outside the home, and the arrival of the new baby. The father said, "I never knew he had so much on his mind." The family decided to engage in some family therapy. The therapy focused on family relationships and on coaching the family to develop a more cooperative relationship with the school, for Bruce's benefit.

This engagement ritual put the decision about family rules regarding talking to outsiders explicitly in the family's hands, thereby eliminating the need for the family to engage in covert solutions to the family–larger system relationship. Once they stopped feeling coerced, they could examine this relationship and make new decisions.

Asking the family to discuss the pros and cons of discussing sensitive issues openly in the family and with an outsider may have a variety of effects. Some families decide not to engage with outside systems at that moment but are able to arrive at this decision in a manner that is overt rather than covert. Other families, like the one in the example above, discover issues among themselves that had been previously hidden by the constraints of the system. Still other families begin to question intergenerational rules regarding interaction with outsiders and make new decisions regarding their relationships with larger systems. This engagement ritual communicates respect to the family, while asking them to become involved in a highly condensed, time-limited journey into their own rules about larger systems.

Transition Rituals to Mark Changes in the Macrosystem

The most difficult transitions for families involve the entry and exit of members, when all relationships must undergo changes. Available relationship options must shift. Similarly, the entrance and exit of members in the family–larger system configuration may pose particular difficulties. Helpers may, in certain cases, have trouble exiting, even when their work is done. Or a family may have a problem in letting go of a particular helper or of help in general. This may be especially salient if the family has endured other losses that have not been adequately dealt with, such that the loss of the helpers becomes metaphorical for other relational losses. The entry of a new helper in a macrosystem where a family has had particular loyalties to a prior helper may be difficult to transact. The family–larger system relationship may need to undergo a transition in the kind of work that is getting done. All of these macrosystemic transitions may be facilitated by rituals. Such rituals, while targeting the macrosystem, are often operating at isomorphic levels, so that developmental transitions between the family and larger systems are also reflections of such transitions within the family. Thus, the need for a "divorce" between a family and a helper may also reflect themes surrounding an actual divorce in the family.

CASE EXAMPLE: THE HELPERS' HANDS ARE TIED

A family–larger system consultation was sought by a family therapy team for two reasons: the family therapist, who had a close relationship with the family, was leaving the area at a time when the family still wanted and required therapy; and the family was embroiled with multiple helpers in a manner that seemed quite confusing and nonproductive (see Figure 5-1).

The family consisted of a single parent, Ms. Aron, and three children, Bud, 18, Kate, 16, and Sam, 14. Another son, 20, had moved out 1 year earlier. In the extended family, the family had endured multiple losses over the previous 2 years, including the separation and divorce of Mr. and Ms. Aron, the death of Ms. Aron's mother, the sudden and unexpected death of Ms. Aron's youngest brother, and the disappearance of Ms. Aron's only other sibling, also a younger brother. Mr. Aaron had moved away and was unavailable to the family. Following the death of Ms. Aron's mother, her father, who had a history of alcoholism, suffered a stroke and had to move to a nursing home.

Presently, the family living in the home included Ms. Aron, Bud, and Kate; Sam was living in a locked facility for delinquent youth, pending a trial for alleged assault on another youngster in the community.

The family was involved with the following larger systems:

1. A family therapy team from a mental health center—including a family therapist, Mr. Marks, and three team members who worked behind a one-way mirror. The family had been referred to this team by social services following an earlier incident involving Sam, which subsequently proved to be an erroneous charge. The family had seen the family therapy team for 4 months.

2. The Department of Social Services—including a social worker who was responsible for securing appropriate services for Sam and the family. In addition, the family was on welfare assistance, following the departure of Mr. Aron.

3. The Juvenile Probation Department—including Sam's probation officer, who was gathering information to present to the court.

4. The public defender's office—including a public defender handling Sam's case.

5. Residential treatment facility—including several workers involved with Sam.

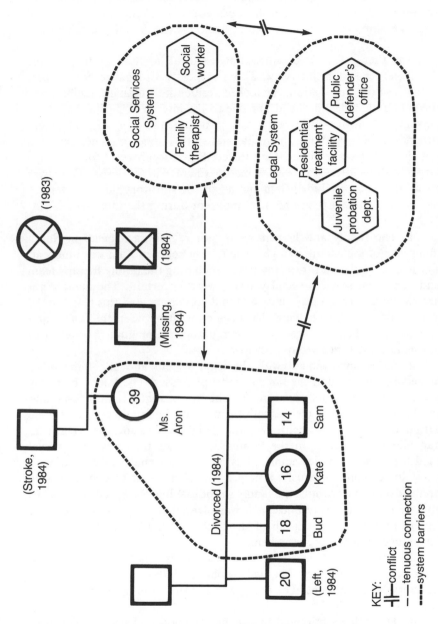

KEY:
—⊦—conflict
− − −tenuous connection
▪▪▪▪system barriers

Figure 5-1. The Aron family genogram and conflicted, tenuous larger–system involvement.

145

6. Public school system—including several special education personnel who had been involved with Sam's educational program for several
years, as Sam had been diagnosed as having severe learning disabilities.

The therapist invited representatives of all of these systems to the
family–larger system interview. Those helpers with legal responsibilities
in the case (i.e., probation, the locked residential treatment facility, and
the public defender) declined to come to the interview, as did the school
personnel. Reasons offered for refusing to come included scheduling and
supervisory advice. Since the residential staff refused to come, Sam was
not allowed to come either. Thus the configuration present for a family–
larger system interview, with a macrosystem whose raison d'etre was
Sam's behavior, excluded Sam and all of the statutory larger systems.

Several salient issues became apparent during the interview.

1. The family and helpers were split regarding a belief in Sam's
innocence of the assault charges. The family believed Sam was innocent.
The helpers gathered for the interview, including the family therapy team
and the social services social worker, were uncertain. The helpers not
present believed Sam was guilty and had communicated this belief to the
family and the other helpers. Thus the conflict between the family and
one group of helpers regarding Sam's innocence or guilt threatened to
triangulate the other group of helpers.

2. Sam's involvement with the legal system and all of the other
helpers followed upon the family's multiple losses. The family had only
one helper in its sphere prior to the charges brought against Sam, and
this helper was about to close with them, since the family appeared to be
getting on its feet. This helper was the social services social worker, who
had taken an interest in the family because of their severe financial
hardship, which was lessening. Thus, in a family that was dealing with
many losses simultaneously, a helper was also about to exit, probably
prematurely, and without the family's input. While the specifics of Sam's
guilt or innocence were unclear, it was clear that Sam had reacted in a
variety of ways following all of the family's losses, and that this had
functioned to bring in many helpers.

3. The family's idea about the helpers was that there were good
helpers and bad helpers. The bad helpers included all of the legal and
statutory larger systems. The only good helpers were the family therapy
team.

4. The helpers mirrored this theme of good and bad helpers, with
each larger system viewing itself and its allies as the good ones, while
viewing the others who did not agree with them as the bad ones. Language used by the helpers in their descriptions was of course more
sophisticated than "good" and "bad," but the message was the same.

5. Rigid boundaries existed among the helpers, who spoke very infrequently to each other. While the family spent a lot of its time with helpers, its boundaries were also very rigid, as the helpers had very little information about the family relationships or issues. The family had developed an interactional style with helpers that involved a lot of noise, but little information. This solution to having a lot of helpers in the family's midst resulted in the helpers often trying to intrude in more ineffective ways. The family described a sense of crisis, a feeling that their family was "falling apart," and the helpers described a sense of helplessness, stating several times throughout the inteview, "Our hands are tied." This metaphor of tied hands reflected both the incredible bureaucracy that was described by the social worker as she spoke of her attempts to get adequate services for Sam, who appeared to be falling through the cracks of several uncoordinated larger systems, and the family therapist's sense that even though the family liked him very much, that liking seemed predicated on not dealing with any of the hard, internal family issues.

6. The family–larger system uproar functioned to deflect focus away from family matters. During the family–larger system interview, the family obliquely indicated that they had many troublesome issues but that there was never any time to deal with these, because of the constant need to deal with the larger systems.

7. A pattern of secrecy seemed to mark the macrosystem at many levels. Several helpers did not come to the interview, not wishing to speak freely in front of the family. The interview itself was divided into several segments, involving differing configurations (i.e., family, social worker, and family therapy team; family therapy team and family; family therapy team). In each segment, information was raised that was being kept secret from those absent. Thus in the first segment, the family and helpers voiced their opinions about the missing helpers and appeared to be getting along with each other. In the second segment, without the social worker, the family raised secret opinions about her that were not evident earlier. In the final segment, the family therapy team raised concerns about the family that they were afraid to raise in the family's presence, including a concern that the family had many secrets. These secrets seemed connected to behavior that had emerged in the family attendant upon their many losses and included veiled references to alcohol problems and sexual acting out. Thus a pattern of secret keeping marked the macrosystem in ways that precluded effective work.

8. The family and family therapy team were facing a developmental transition that mirrored family issues regarding loss and members leaving. While the leaving of a therapist is certainly not of the magnitude of the leaving of a family member, this family drew a lot of comparisons. Ms. Aron spoke of sudden and unexpected losses of family members and compared this to prior therapists they had had, who left without telling them.

She spoke of children leaving home in a prepared and expected way and compared this to their current family therapist telling them he was leaving. Family members also compared the family therapist and the son, Sam, calling them both the "glue that held the family together." It appeared that the pending loss of Sam because of the court charges and the leaving of the therapist had become fused in the minds of family members. For the family therapist and his team, this designation of being the glue that held the family together seemed to make doing effective work even more difficult.

A ritual intervention was designed to address the family and family therapist subsystem of the macrosystem. This was done for several reasons. It was the family therapist who had asked for the consultation. The lack of involvment of many of the other systems was taken as an indication that to attempt to intervene at that level could, in fact, be resented and make things worse. Certain constraints in the macrosystem were judged to be statutory and unamenable to intervention presently. Finally, since patterns in the family and between the family and the family therapy team appeared to be isomorphic with patterns in the entire macrosystem, it was felt that intervention in the most available subsystem might have reverberating effects.

The intervention focused on the potential benefits of expected and planned-for leavings and losses, highlighting the leaving of the family therapist as an opportunity to "ask the unasked questions and receive the unanswered answers." The two children living at home, Bud and Kate, were asked to make a question box that would hold everyone's questions. The members of the family and the family therapist and his team were asked to each write down one question that they would like answered before the current therapy ended. These were to be anonymous questions, placed in sealed envelopes. Ms. Aron was asked to see if it would be possible to have Sam at the next session. If this was not possible, she was asked to collect a question from him. Members of the family and the family therapy team were told to take turns taking questions out of the box, in order to free the family therapist from the potential position of the messenger bringing the bad news. Family members and team members, including the therapist, were also told to take turns going behind the one-way mirror in order to help the team deepen and broaden the questions. This was suggested because family members seemed very expert at cueing each other in the room, because using the mirror and team in this fashion has been shown to be an efficacious intervention in families with secrets that preclude effective work (see Chapter 6, "A 40-year secret," case involving this intervention), and because this paved the way for the therapist's pending exit from the family.

This intervention prepared the family and family therapist subsystem for an in-session ritual that would utilize the next sessions in a very unusual and unexpected way capable of altering stuck patterns. Prior to the prescription, the family therapist and team felt they had only one position available to them, which was to support the family against all the bad helpers. Although the family appreciated this support, it obviated against effective family therapy. Since the family regarded the family therapist and the team as members of the family, the consultant's directions utilized this and prescribed a system that put family members and the family therapy team on the same level by asking them all to do the same thing, bring an unanswered question. The team's position vis-à-vis the family before the consultation was thus highlighted without ever pointing to it openly in a way that might scold or criticize. The box was requested in order to communicate symbolically that the questions and answers could be contained and not overwhelm people, which seemed to be a covert fear. The issue of the loss of the therapist was utilized as a metaphor for other family losses, which had previously been too difficult to deal with and which seemed to be exquisitely related to the family's current problems. Thus the developmental transition in the macrosystem, the therapist's leaving, provided a vehicle for other changes.

The intervention could free the family therapist from a stuck position, allowing him to elaborate his remaining work with the family without the prior constraints. Topics could be raised that were previously off limits. The position of the therapist and team as "family members" could shift and the hands of the family therapist and team could be untied.

Identity Redefinition Rituals

Certain individuals and families obtain identities by virtue of their involvement with larger systems. This is particularly true when labels have been used repeatedly by the larger systems in reference to the family or individual members, and such labels have come to totalize the family and reduce its complexity. A family may become known as an "anorexic" or a "psychotic" family, or an individual family member may become known as a "compulsive handwasher" or a "school phobic." While such labels may have their efficacy in certain circumstances, they often function in ways that limit perceptions and narrow solution choices. The labeled identity of an individual or a family frequently occurs when larger systems such as schools or medical systems are continually involved in the family's life. Here differences between the family and larger systems are often submerged, and unquestioned labels come to calibrate the relationships within the family and between the family and larger systems. Particular behavior that the label identifies becomes affirmed and predictable. Other options become constrained and unavailable. Rituals to redefine identities may be useful when the therapist or consultant discerns that labels have come to totalize complex human beings.

BRIEF EXAMPLE: FROM "MALINGERERS" TO "SURVIVORS"

A couple was referred to therapy by a veteran's hospital. The husband, 48, had injured his back in the armed services 20 years earlier, shortly after the couple married. This back injury required him to interact with medical systems, including physicians and a physical therapist. Over the years, an unusual cycle developed in which the husband's back would improve and he would disengage from larger systems and return to work until the next time his back would go out. While he was feeling well, he and his wife had a fairly positive relationship. During this time, the husband would work. At some point, usually after 6 or 8 months, the wife would notice her husband not taking care of himself. He would stop his exercise and begin to overeat and gain weight. She would become angry and withdraw from him. His back would go out, and he would become disabled once again, requiring the entry of larger systems. Since this cycle had occurred many times, the husband was considered a malingerer by larger systems and by his wife. Both tended to treat him with angry responses. During times when his back was out, which would last several months, the wife would seek help from therapists. When the husband's physical condition improved, the wife would disengage from the therapy relationships. Several therapists had encouraged her to leave her husband, since he became extremely demanding and tyrannical during the periods of his incapacitation. Just as medical personnel viewed the husband as malingering, so therapists viewed the wife as unable or unwilling to act in her own behalf. The messages to the couple from larger systems who interacted with them during difficult times were largely negative. No one explored what went on for the couple during the periods when the husband's health improved and they were disengaged from larger systems.

At the beginning of the couple's therapy, this cycle was explored. Rather than focusing on the time of the cycle when the husband was disabled and the wife was despairing, the therapist chose to focus on how the couple emerged from this period each time, on what strengths were mobilized, on what prevented them from simply giving up. The therapist framed them as survivors, rather than as malingerers, and asked them to embark on an exploration of survivorhood in order to build on that aspect of their relationship. The couple and the larger systems had never viewed their situation from this perspective. The husband was asked to interview his wife in order to gain her perspective on his strengths, and the wife was asked to interview her husband in order to gain his perspecting on her strengths. Together with the therapist, they fashioned a report to larger systems on the ways they would like to be worked with in the future, to enhance their position as survivors rather than as malingerers. This process took several months, during which time the husband was able to maintain his exercise regime, rather than abandoning it as he always had before. The cycles between husband and wife, and between the couple and helpers, shifted, such that anger and distancing were no longer utilized when the husband again had some trouble with his back.

The entire therapy focused on presenting the couple with a new identity vis-à-vis each other and larger systems. A dramatic ritual celebrating survivorship, in which the couple videotaped a history of their struggles and how they had overcome these, terminated the therapy.

It is important when utilizing identity-redefinition rituals to carefully analyze the position of the other larger systems regarding the issue of labels. Here one seeks to avoid insulting the other larger systems in ways that might ultimately harm the family. Terms like "experiment" or "pretend" are often useful in securing the cooperation of other systems. Once a label is dropped, even experimentally, members of the macrosystem are usually able to see the new and more complex behavior that becomes available. (See "From 'hyperactive' to 'normal but naughty'," Chapter 6, for a case utilizing an identity redefinition ritual.)

Time Division/Message Distinction Rituals

Several years ago, the original Milan team described an intervention that they called a "ritualized prescription: odd days and even days" (Selvini Palazzoli *et al.*, 1978b). This ritual was intended for two-parent families with a symptomatic child, when the therapist had discerned that the child was the recipient of simultaneous and contradictory messages from the parents.

When a family is engaged with multiple larger systems, it is not unusual for it to be the recipient of simultaneous and contradictory ideas from the various helpers, resulting in confusion or paralysis of action. One family member may also find that he or she is the recipient of such simultaneous and contradictory messages from other family members and helpers (see the case example in Chapter 4, "The more help, the more helplessness"). The time division/message distinction ritual is intended for these occasions. The family, alone or with helpers, is invited to divide the week and assign particular messages to specific days. For instance, a family may be hearing from one helper that the etiology of a problem and its only solution is internal, while hearing from another helper that the etiology of that same problem and its only solution is interactional. The family may be asked to believe and act on one point of view for half the week and on the other point of view for half the week. This would, of course, require specific actions vis-à-vis the larger systems as well. The family may be asked to engage with particular larger systems on certain days or to give particular messages to helpers on certain days, as in the case discussed in Chapter 4, "The more help, the more helplessness." The ritual utilizes time and condensed dramatization of divergent points of view while putting the family in charge of decisions, thereby interdicting the escalating complementarity that frequently marks the relationship between family and helpers when contradictory points of view are presented to the family and the family exhibits more and more confusion.

Termination Rituals

Some families have a difficult time disengaging from larger systems and owning their own changes and a sense of their own resources. This is particularly true for families who have had to interact with larger systems over a long period of time, because of the illness or handicap of a member or long-term financial hardship. Here a termination ritual, which clearly marks the family's autonomous functioning and celebrates its own resources, may be in order.

CASE EXAMPLE: THE POTATO AND THE KIWI FRUIT

In Chapter 2, the Moore family was described as born with helpers. The family formed with outside systems in its midst because of the congenital heart problems of the firstborn, Sandra. When Sandra's heart problems were surgically repaired, the family began to interact with helpers regarding Sandra's unusual eating preferences for french fries, bread, and milk. All family relationships in the nuclear family, with the extended family and with helpers were calibrated by this problem.

By the end of the family therapy, many relationships had changed. For the first time in 12 years the family was going to be a family without helpers. A termination ritual, utilizing the symbols of the therapy and highlighting the family's strengths and resources, was given to the family at the last therapy session. This session was a celebration meal brought by the family, dramatically illustrating the changes in the family.

At the end of the meal, the therapist said to the family, "You've brought food to me a couple of times, so tonight I want to give something to you." Here the more symmetrical relationship existing at the end of therapy was highlighted. The therapist then took a potato and a kiwi fruit out of a bag and placed them on the table. Sandra laughed. The therapist said, "You know what that is," and Sandra replied with disgust, "Kiwi fruit." All laughed. The therapist said, "And you know what that is," and Sandra said brightly, "Potato!" The therapist then asked, "Why do you think I brought these?" Mr. Moore, teasing, said, "Because Sandra likes both?" Sandra immediately retorted, "No way, I hate kiwi!" All laughed. The therapist said, "Well, first of all, they're not to eat. Obviously, the potato wouldn't be too good to eat like that, huh?" Here Sandra interjected, "We could cook it!" Family members, who previously were enormously upset by Sandra's love of potatoes, simply laughed.

The therapist continued, "I brought them I guess, in terms of some of the things we've been working on. I remember way back in the first session when we got together, Sandra said the dietician wanted her to eat kiwi fruit and she hated it. I asked how it was, and she said, 'yucch, awful!' But potatoes have been something that all along you really liked. And you still do, hmmm. (Sandra replied, 'Yes'.) So, it seems to me that the potato and the kiwi fruit represent the thing that you like and the things that you really don't like. Okay, as well I think, as I thought about it, it's one way to think about the difficulties that the family got into, where some things got pretty stuck around preferences, likes, dislikes, kind of normal things getting out of hand. Some things got pretty out of hand, so that your relationship (*indicating the mother and Sandra*) really suffered, and the two of you (*indicating the mother and father*) were struggling over this.

"So I brought this, not for you to eat, but for you to take home, and what I'd like you to do with these is for Sandra and Ellen, with your folks around, to take them and put them in a big plastic bowl, fill the bowl with water and put them in the freezer. Put them in the back of the freezer, so you'll have them. They will be there, Okay. Now, the reason I want you to do that is I think there will be times in the life of the family in the future when the family may be unsure how to solve a particular problem. It might be difficult to decide if something is a big problem, whether something is simply a matter of personal preference, an expression of individual development, or whether what's going on is a serious problem for an individual, a problem for two people, a problem for the whole family. When you find yourselves in that kind of quandary, what I would like to recommend that you do is take the potato and kiwi fruit out of the freezer, let them thaw out, and have a family discussion as to whether it is a problem the family can handle on its own, whether you need a hand with it, whether it is just a matter of things being individual preferences, or whether it is individual growth and development that the family is experiencing with her (*Sandra*) getting older, her (*Ellen*) becoming a teenager, the two of you aging as a couple (*parents laugh*). For instance, Ellen may decide to become very stubborn. She may decide to imitate Sandra, or she may decide to do something more original than that, or Sandra may decide to go out with some boys the parents do not like (*Sandra laughs with delight*), or the two of you may be unable to resolve an issue, or there may be some struggles with extended family—things that are normal for families to go through. So, what I am recommending is that at those times any one of you could initiate thawing out the potato and the kiwi fruit and that is a sign to have a family discussion and to make some decisions, maybe make some new decisions. The two of you are good at that, from what I experienced. You came in and told me how you wanted to work. You developed a plan. You carried it out. So then afterwards you can freeze it again, and that will be yours for as long as you want it."

Here the family thanked the therapist, took the potato and the kiwi fruit, and left. In a 6-month follow-up by mail, the family stated they were doing well and there was no symptomatic behavior.

This termination ritual highlighted the family's resources in a number of ways, at a point when they were terminating a 12-year involvement with larger systems. It reframed all of the difficulties around Sandra's unusual eating as that which will now provide opportunities for the family to handle problems. Future problems were cast in the frame of normal, developmental, expectable, and solvable. Future involvement with helpers was listed as a possible, but not required, option. Family connectedness was highlighted, while individual initiative was also maintained. Humor permeated the entire ritual. Therapy and the family's relationship to larger systems was terminated with symbols of the entire therapy remaining with the family "in the back of the freezer," thus available, but not necessary, in a daily way (Imber-Black, 1986c).

Termination rituals are especially useful when the relationship between family and larger systems has been ultimately positive and both family and helpers are having difficulty letting go of each other. Many relationships in our culture have prescribed rituals for endings and mutual expression of appreciation. The relationship between clients and public-sector helpers is a notable exception. Each may go in search of new problems to maintain the relationship. A simple termination ritual that facilitates expression of appreciation and marks a clear ending is one in which client and helper give a small gift to each other that symbolizes hopes for the future. Such gifts are best either made or consisting of an item already belonging to the giver. This obviates against financial concerns and contributes to the sought-after expression of symmetry in the relationship, which the ritual intends.

POSTSESSION INTERVENTION

Following assessment of the family–larger system relationship, certain interventions may be generated that are not delivered at the end of a session but are sent after a session or are part of ongoing work after such assessment. These include memos, reports, coaching, and advocacy. Coaching and advocacy will be discussed in Chapter 6 in an examination of ongoing relationships with larger systems.

Following a family–larger system interview, a consultant may wish to communicate his or her ideas to all who were present by the use of a memo. There are several reasons to utilize a memo in this way. Memos are familiar symbols to helpers. When a memo is sent to the family and helpers, an implicit message is also sent that both comments on the value of shared and open information in the macrosystem and draws a temporary boundary around all the participants, delineating them as members of a macrosystem. Memos are an especially useful way to communicate ideas when there are missing members who are important in the macrosystem but, for one reason or another, have not come to the interview, or who may have left early. Finally, sending a memo to the family members and the helpers is usually an unexpected event, whose effect may therefore be to impart information through unexpectedness.

Since a consultant is generally brought in by one helper, the memo may be sent directly to that person, with a covering letter requesting that copies of the memo be sent to all of the participants. In this way, the consultant removes himself or herself from ongoing relatedness to the macrosystem.

CASE EXAMPLE: IF ONE HELPER IS GOOD, MORE MUST BE BETTER

A family–larger system interview was requested by a family therapist. The interview included Mr. and Mrs. Brandon, both 35, Helen, the identified patient, 16, Bob, 14, the family therapist, the father's individual therapist, and Helen's probation officer, who was next planning to bring in for Helen a counselor specializing in sexuality. Helen had been a "good girl" until adolescence. Her difficulties were contained within the family and included such things as fighting with the parents, until 8 months earlier when she used her father's checks and he pressed charges against her, thus initiating the entry of outside systems into the family sphere. A pattern quickly developed, of identifying new problems in the girl and involving new specialists to solve the problems. Each so-called resolution was countered by a new symptom, leading to the entry of a new expert. The family–larger system interview focused on this pattern.

During the course of the interview, four major relational areas were explored. The first involved alliances in the ecosystem.

CONSULTANT: Who has been the most helpful in working on these problems?

FATHER: Everyone. They've all helped . . . each in their own way.

HELEN: The probation officer has been most helpful to my father.

CONSULTANT: How?

HELEN: He turns to her for support.

CONSULTANT: Does he turn to her before turning to anyone else?

HELEN: Yes, he talks to her before anyone, before my mother.

Further questions illuminated a countervailing alliance between Mrs. Brandon and the family therapist. Mr. Brandon had recently formed another alliance with his individual therapist. Bob added that the parents had been helped the most by the outsiders. A picture began to emerge in which problems posed by the girl resulted in the generation of support for the parents and an escalating symmetrical pattern of each parent getting more and more assistance from outsiders.

Second, optimism and pessimism of the outside helpers were explored, and a pattern was revealed in which new outsiders entered the family sphere with great hope and enthusiasm and were warmly welcomed by the parents. Comfortable, nonchallenging relationships, marked by support and understanding, developed quickly. After a few months each helper grew pessimistic, identified a new problem, and enlisted a new helper.

The third area explored beliefs about the future and the efficacy of professional help.

CONSULTANT: What do you think the picture will be 5 years from now for Helen?

MOTHER: Oh, she'll be fine.

CONSULTANT: How will she do it? With help? On her own?

FATHER: She'll do it alone. Hard knocks. She's stubborn. The more help you give her, the more she doesn't want it!

FAMILY THERAPIST: I think she'll have some hard times and then she'll do all right. I think her parents will have an easier time with Bob.

BOB: I think she's gonna do just fine. And without professional help.

HELEN: It'll be sooner than 5 years. And I'm going to do it on my own!

During this brief interchange, the various outside professionals appeared quite surprised.

The interview per se had the impact of intervention, since information was generated regarding relationships the present function of Helen's behavior in the ecosystem, and the "more of the same" pattern. The consultant then pulled all this together in two interventions. The first was delivered as an opinion to all of the participants and positively reframed Helen's behavior as that which "brought home parents for her parents." Thus, the place of outsiders was framed as helpful and necessary, but not for work on Helen's problems. Helen was informed by the consultant that her parents would be the best judges of how many helpers they needed and for how long, and that she could "take a vacation" from that job. She responded immediately, "I plan to, starting now!" In addition to elaborating on the function of Helen's problems in the ecosystem, this comment framed the parents as more openly in charge of their relationship to helpers, as consumers of service rather than as participants in a comfortable and covert symmetry.

The following day the consultant sent a memo to the family therapist, with copies to all participants in the interview.

To: Dr. Allen   Date: December 1984
From: Dr. Evan Imber-Black   Re: The Brandon Family

I am writing in follow-up to the consultation I did with you, the Brandon family, Ms. Reilly (probation officer), and Dr. Larkin (individual therapist). I would like to make the following recommendation to you, based on information gathered in the session. Since the family members agreed that Helen will eventually improve and succeed in life on her own without professional input, since all seemed to agree with Mr. Brandon that the more helpers that attempt to help Helen, the more determined she is to make it on her own, and since it was the consensus of those present that the rest of the family, particularly Mr. and Mrs. Brandon, have benefited from their interactions with helping professionals, I would recommend that you continue to see the family, but that Helen not be allowed to attend such sessions. This will both assist the family and provide the only fair test of the belief that Helen will improve her life without professional helpers.

cc: The Brandon Family
    Ms. Reilly
    Dr. Larkin

Following the session and receipt of the memo, the probation officer remarked, "I found out I'm working harder than this family. I'm not going to do that anymore!"

At the first family therapy session following this interview, Bob, who had ordinarily refused to participate verbally and often slept at sessions, very excitedly told the therapist that his parents, who had previously presented a united front, were actively fighting with one another. The therapist was allowed to focus on their marital relationship for the first time. Follow-up information collected 3 months after this consulting interview indicated that the parents continued in therapy with a clear contract to work on their own relationship, holding sessions in which Helen's name was not even mentioned. The family had trimmed its list of helpers, and the probation officer was working to maintain clear boundaries vis-à-vis other shared cases. Most recently, the parents reported experiencing positive interactions with Helen for the first time in 2 years, and Helen was reported to have said, "I told you I could do it on my own" (Imber Coppersmith, 1983).

Here the memo served to further elaborate the notion that the family and helpers were all in the same boat and that there existed the possibility of arranging treatment in a very different fashion.

A memo may also be a useful tool when lines are drawn sharply in the macrosystem and anger is high between family and helpers.

BRIEF EXAMPLE: MEDIATING THE FAMILY–LARGER SYSTEM RELATIONSHIP

In Chapter 1, the "History repeats itself" case described a family and a residential treatment facility at war with each other. Each saw the other side as uncooperative, unwilling to work, and so on. Their shared member, the family's daughter, Corey, was deteriorating as the war between the family and the residence escalated. All did agree, however, to attend a family–larger system interview. The parents sat on one side of the room, while the residential staff sat on the other. Corey sat in the middle. It was extremely difficult for conversations to ensue. Gradually, each side described its anger, disappointments, and extreme frustration. The macrosystem was beset by escalating symmetry, as the family and the helpers each insisted on their point of view prevailing. Neither side was able to hear the other, and disqualification was high. During the course of the interview, the consultant began to assume a mediator's role, searching for small indications of willingness to compromise in return for getting part of what each side wanted. Gradually, a few halting indications were made that each side might give in a little, if they saw movement on the other side. The symmetrical pattern began to be available in the service of what was framed as a fresh start. Following the interview, the consultant sent her opinions in a memo to the residential director who had requested the consultation and asked that copies be sent to all who were present.

To: Director
Re: The Residential Staff and the Franklin Family Consultation

Thank you for the opportunity to meet with you, the family, your staff, and others concerned in this case. I would like to offer the following conclusions based on our interview together.

It seems to me that all concerned have been working very hard in this situation. Despite obvious frustration and conflict on both sides, I feel optimistic that people on both sides of the issue were willing to sit down and discuss the matter in an attempt to make a fresh start on Corey's behalf.

Further, I was impressed that both the family therapist and the cottage manager recognize the need for a fresh start regarding family sessions and are willing to step aside at this moment in the service of exploring a fresh start.

Since mistrust had been high on both sides before our meeting, I would recommend small steps and slow steps in order to determine the best way to build a useful working relationship between the family and the residence.

To facilitate this, I suggest that the family begin having sessions with you. If possible, these sessions should be weekly for at least six or eight sessions. Later, these may be spaced out a bit more. The first four sessions should be spent building a foundation and might focus on gaining a deeper understanding of the parents, their families of origin, and any and all present concerns. These early sessions should *not* deal with the sexual abuse issue, nor should they deal with the parents' desire to have their daughter home on visits. In other words, I am suggesting that each side demonstrate willingness to postpone their most important issue in the spirit of carefully constructing a new relationship. Both the family and the therapist should candidly evaluate these sessions and give feedback to each other on the quality of the session, during the last 10 minutes.

Following these four sessions, I suggest a format that alternates who decides the topics for discussion. Thus, at the end of the fourth session, the family and the therapist could flip a coin to determine who will go first. If the family wins the toss, they will determine the topic for the next session. At the following session, the therapist will determine the topic, and so on. If a session is missed, for whatever reason, the next session will remain with the topic for the missed session. In this way, the diverse and sometimes conflictual needs of the family and the center will be given equal time and energy. The last 10 minutes should remain as feedback.

Since a major concern to the family seems to be private visits and a major concern of the residence seems to be Corey's safety, I also suggest beginning half-hour unsupervised visits on campus. The success of such visits can be discussed and their length negotiated in family sessions. However, in order to free Corey from the position of being like a child caught between divorced parents, it is crucial that the parents agree not to discuss the residence treatment, and so on, during these visits, *and* that the staff agree not to ask Corey what she discussed with her parents during these visits. In other words, even though mistrust has been very high, each side needs to pretend to trust, at least a little bit, in order to establish a fresh start.

This interview and the memo had the effect of providing an opportunity for a new and different sort of relationship between the residence and the family. The instructions in the memo, utilizing an odd session–even session format, were designed to utilize the existing symmetry in the macrosystem but to offer different content for the pattern. While the relationship between the family and the residence never became a wonderful one, it did become a working one in which Corey was freed from her previously triangulated position.

Memos should be phrased carefully, utilizing language that both the professionals and the family will understand. Familiar phrases from the interview may be usefully repeated in the memo. The memo may offer suggestions for delineating helpers' roles, instructions for rituals, paradoxical prescriptions of the macrosystem, or some careful combination of these. Memos should always communicate respect for the participants and should *not* utilize sarcasm.

REPORTS AS INTERVENTIONS

Many families who are engaged with larger systems over a long period of time become used to having reports written about them. Such reports are frequently read as the totalized truth about a family or a situation, rather than as a subjective viewpoint. If a family is chronically involved with large public-sector systems such as welfare, such reports form part of the ongoing helper–helpee complementarity, since the family is always the subsystem being written about and is never in the position of writer. When these conditions pertain, a therapist working with the family may wish to invite the family to write their own report and to submit it along with other reports that have been written.

BRIEF EXAMPLE: WHY DON'T THEY SAY IT IN PLAIN ENGLISH?

A family consisting of a mother, stepfather, and son was involved with public-sector systems for many years regarding many problems. Both parents came from families that had also been chronically involved with outside systems, and each parent had lived a major portion of childhood in foster care. At the time of the referral for family therapy, the son, now a teenager, had been removed from the home and was living in a group home because of delinquent behavior. The parents were seeking to obtain his return to their custody, and a court hearing was pending. In the first interview, during which the family therapist obtained a history of the parents' relationship with helpers, it became apparent that all of their previous relationships with helpers had been problematic and unsuccessful. They had entered family therapy because they felt coerced to do so in order to get their son back. Problems between the family and helpers seemed also to function to prevent resolution of family issues, including alcohol problems of the stepfather. This initial focus on the family's relationship with helpers seemed to engage the family, as this was a very different focus than what they were used to from helpers.

At the start of the second session, the mother began by asking the family therapist, "What's a character disorder?" When the therapist investigated the meaning of the mother's question, the mother stated that the family had just seen a report, written about them by a psychologist for the court, that stated that the mother had a character disorder. The mother then said, "I don't know what it means—I only know it can't be something good!" The therapist proceeded to explain what is generally meant by the term, and the mother replied, "Well, why don't they say it in plain English." The parents then began to tell the therapist that they had frequently had reports written about them and that most often the reports were very negative, ignored any of their strengths, and were hard to understand.

The family therapist proposed to the family that they write their own report and submit it to the court along with the reports of professionals that were being submitted. She indicated that she did not know if their report would have a big impact on the outcome of their case but that likely it would show their sincerity. She suggested that she and the family actually cocreate a report that would focus on family strengths, their problems and struggles, and their experiences with larger systems. The parents became very enthusiastic, and the stepfather remarked, "You know, I don't know if this will make any difference to the judge, but it makes a difference to me—this is the first time anybody's asked us what we think."

The next three sessions were spent developing the report. The parents worked hard on it together at home and remarked that this was the first time that they didn't feel split by the stresses of dealing with outside systems. They were clear about their strengths and candid about their existing problems. The stepfather both owned his alcohol problem and became willing to work on it in therapy. They submitted the report to the court and remarked to the therapist that they had stopped feeling so victimized by the larger systems.

While they did not get their son back at this first court hearing, he was returned 6 months later. During the 6 months, the parents worked very hard with the family therapist and formed a positive relationship with an outside helper for the first time in their lives. The report became on ongoing tool in the therapy, as the family and the therapist continually updated the report so that it became a vivid marker for therapeutic change.

Cocreated reports may also be used at the end of work with a family who has had long-standing relationships with outside systems. As such the report becomes a kind of termination ritual and may include a ritualized signing by all concerned. The family is given a copy for their own keeping, thus communicating a more symmetrical relationship replacing the former helper–helpee complementarity.

The report intervention functions to shift the family from the rigid position of client to the level of helper to themselves. It is interesting to note that in many applications of this intervention, not one family has lied, dissembled, or chosen to omit an honest appraisal of their difficulties from the report.

CONCLUSION

Family–larger system interventions call upon a therapist's or consultant's acumen and creativity. Care must be taken to design interventions that provide new information and enhance the well-being and empowerment of the participants in the macrosystem. While predictability is never absolute in human systems, interventions that are anchored in respect, careful multilevel assessment and an abiding belief in the interconnection and interdependence of people comprising a macrosystem are likely to have effective outcomes.

CHAPTER 6

Creating a New Relationship between a Family and Larger Systems: Ongoing Work

Certain families are required to interact with larger systems and multiple helpers over significant portions of their life cycle. This requirement may be due to the presence of severe or chronic illness that necessitates ongoing involvement with medical facilities and personnel, developmental disabilities that may demand involvement with both medical and educational systems, or poverty that requires interaction with the welfare system and all of its adjuncts in housing, food, health care, and employment. Thus those already most stressed in our society by illness, poverty, or both generally have the additional stress of dealing with larger systems.

The larger systems rarely, if ever, have a view of their work that conceptualizes issues about families and complex systems. Medical and educational systems generally view their mandates as on behalf of individuals. Interaction with families may be required, but this is not seen as the heart of the matter and is often seen as a necessary evil. The welfare system in our culture, while ostensibly organized to support families, in fact frequently fragments them through practices and policies that lack appreciation both of diverse family forms and of the impact of interventions on delicate family ecologies.

When families are required to interact with larger systems, the family–larger system relationship is seldom regarded as a salient dimension by either family or larger system and tends to become invisible. When attended to at all, each family–larger system interaction is viewed as special or unique, reflecting the idiosyncracies of an individual family member and one or two helpers, or of a whole family that gets labeled as difficult.

Work with families who *must* interact with larger systems for long portions of their life cycle calls upon additional and sometimes different assumptions and skills in the therapist than work with families who have become stuck with larger systems due to unfortunate interactional patterns.

COMMON THEMES

When families and larger systems *must* interact with each other, certain common themes frequently emerge.

The family system and the larger system often hold emotional and physical *survival* value for one or more family members. Issues of loss of a member, a relationship, or ability to function loom. In the case of chronic or life-threatening illness, conflict between the family and larger systems may create triangles of special proportions. Threats to exclude the shared member by either system or threats to withdraw needed services or required relationships may keep the macrosystem precariously balanced at the point of impending crisis. Interactions between the family and the larger system are frequently intense and thus stressful.

The family therapist who enters this macrosystem must be cognizant of this issue of survival and must frequently work hard to avoid being caught up in the framework of intensity and crisis, while simultaneously demonstrating an understanding of the serious nature of the issues.

The family system and the larger systems seldom share enough *information* with each other. Since the larger systems most frequently interact with only one member of the family, many aspects of a family's circumstances never become available or clear. Judgments are made and acted upon with incomplete information. Families' particular ways of imparting and processing information are often ignored or misunderstood. The working methods of the larger systems are often not explained, and families are expected to discern the rules and comply. Careful explanation of the reasons for decisions, policy changes, or referrals may not be given, may be given in language that a family does not understand, or may be given clearly, but at a time when a family is experiencing too much stress to hear clearly. Many families lack the skills to inquire, including knowing what questions or whom to ask. A sense of helplessness may turn into anger, leading rapidly to further distancing by the larger system. Lacking specific information, both families and larger systems tend to fill in what's missing with their own fantasies, which, when acted upon, may lead to further misunderstanding. The family therapist may function here as a translator, assisting a family in negotiations with larger systems.

When a family is required to interact with larger systems for long periods of time, the *boundaries* of the family must shift, sometimes profoundly, in order to accommodate the continual presence of larger systems. The line between private and public becomes blurred for such families, as far more of the family's internal business becomes known in the larger system.

A family's particular history and experience with larger systems is a salient aspect of the boundary issue. If a family has been very private, isolated, or otherwise disengaged from large formal systems and is suddenly required to interact with a hospital or a welfare department, that family may have an especially difficult time. Lacking skills in their repertoire for dealing with larger systems, such a family may initially attempt to distance. Such distancing may be easily misunderstood as lack of interest in an ill member or inability to cope with internal family matters, rather than an initial inability to alter boundaries in order to accommodate the demands of the larger system. If, as often happens, the larger system distances in turn, then a macrosystem marked by rigid boundaries may develop.

The boundaries between families and larger systems that exist over long periods of time frequently show an unusual combination of diffusion and rigidity. Families may be required to share much more information with the larger system than the larger system is required to share with the family. The door to the family system may be forced to be open to multiple helpers in order to receive needed services, while the door to the larger systems will be highly regulated by formal and complex processes.

The family therapist must be cognizant of this skewed boundary and may coach the family in ways to gain necessary access to the larger system, while simultaneously shoring up family boundaries from inappropriate intrusion.

In order to deal with the presence of larger systems over a long period of time, many families "appoint" one member to do most of the interaction with the larger system. This person becomes the *conduit* between the family and the larger system. The larger system may make the error of assuming that this person is also the major decision maker for the family, when in fact she (the conduit is most often the mother) may simply be the message carrier between the systems. This conduit role is a difficult and stressful one, requiring the translation of messages between the family and larger systems.

Larger systems often utilize this conduit, while at the same time designating this person as overinvolved. It is important for the family therapist to assess this person's position in the macrosystem and utilize planful alliances, while reducing the stress placed on a single individual.

SPECIAL PROBLEMS: LABELING, STIGMA, AND SECRECY

The issues that generally bring families into contact with larger systems for protracted periods of time tend to include particular obstacles to development and change, including labeling, stigma, and secrecy.

Labeling

When a person, a family, or a condition is labeled, certain options for behavior may become available, while other options become totally unavailable. That the label and the behavior it implies are culturally determined is immediately forgotten, in favor of a point of view that understands the label as "truth." Labels express social norms and ideologies but are seldom seen from this perspective. Sarason and Doris (1979), in a discussion of the label "mental retardation," state, "Mental retardation is never a thing or a characteristic of an individual but rather a social invention stemming from time-bound societal values and ideology that makes diagnosis and management seem both necessary and socially desirable. The shifting definitions and management of mental retardation are not understandable in terms of the 'essence' of the 'condition' but rather in terms of changing social values and conditions" (p. 417).

Certain larger systems will gain permission to become involved in a case depending on the label involved. Thus, a mental health system will enter if a truant boy is labeled "depressed," while a probation system may enter if that same boy is labeled "delinquent."

Labels calibrate relationships, both within families and between families and larger systems. When the family and the larger system disagree about a particular label, then conflict will likely ensue. The family may go in search of other larger systems or of its own solutions. This is particularly the case when finances are involved, as when a family and a school system are in conflict regarding the appropriate label for a child, when such labeling is linked to required educational services. This sort of argument over labels becomes particularly important for the family therapist accepting referrals from larger systems, since the manner of accepting the referral can easily ally the therapist with the larger system before any assessment can be made. If a school refers a family for family therapy rather than providing special educational services to a child whom the family and physician are labeling developmentally disabled, and a family therapist blindly takes the referral without first assessing the conflict over labeling, he or she will be seen by the family as the school's ally.

Conversely, when the family and the larger systems are in total agreement regarding a label, the macrosystem tends to reify, and creative interventions for development and change are extinguished. When one member of a family is labeled by outside systems, other members often develop their own labels, constraining their identities both within the family and in the macrosystem. This phenomenon and its change is shown in the following case.

CASE EXAMPLE: FROM "HYPERACTIVE" TO "NORMAL BUT NAUGHTY"

The Taylor family, consisting of a mother, Ann, a father, Paul, and their 11-year-old daughter, Gina, was referred for family therapy by a pediatrician who had been treating Gina for hyperactivity since age 3. Physicians, school personnel, and family members all agreed with the label hyperactive, and Gina had been taking Ritalin for 8 years. The term "hyperactive" was the preferred explanation for any and all behavior of Gina by the medical, school, and family systems. Family, school, and physician were joined in a medical diagnosis and treatment of the girl's behavior. Other efforts, such as limit setting or discipline, were not employed. The referral for family therapy came because Gina's behavior had been worsening *and* she was fast approaching an age when the medication would have to be stopped. The father was a skilled laborer; the mother did not work outside the home. Their extended families lived within commuting distance, but visits were infrequent because the grandparents refused to cope with the girl's often outrageous behavior. The entire family, including the identified patient, were united in their reference to the girl as hyperactive. Both parents reported increasing frustration, however, with the recent escalation of the girl's behavior, citing her tantrums, fights in school, refusal to listen, gluing of drawers shut on furniture, and placing of peanut butter in family members' clothing as among their chief complaints. The family agreed that Gina was worse when Ann was alone with her than when both parents were present and that Ann would relate her difficulties with the girl to Paul when he came home. The child was thus the intense focus of discussion between her parents. Both parents verbally agreed that the girl's problem was hyperactivity; however, Paul occasionally revealed his growing disenchantment with this point of view. When pushed a bit by the therapist in the first session to consider other formulations, Paul quickly backed off and deferred to his wife. He said he occasionally lost his temper with Gina but would then feel enormously guilty, because she was hyperactive. This label and the family's belief system about what it implied prevented the parents from searching for new solutions. By the time they entered therapy, the family appeared exhausted and frightened about the future. The parents, while ostensibly united regarding the girl, showed covert conflict at an analogic level. It could not be determined whether such conflict existed before Gina's symptoms, which then might have served as an unfortunate solution to bring the parents together, or whether the conflict came as a result of trying to handle the girl with no success. What was apparent, however, was that marital issues existed that could not be openly discussed.

At the first session the therapy team discovered that the family had been intensely involved with a variety of medical and school personnel for many years regarding Gina. There was no one person with whom any family member was allied. Rather, the parents looked to these systems to define the problem and by and large followed the lead of experts with respect to their child. Both parents expressed doubt that they, as parents, knew the right thing to do. Over the years many different professionals had interacted with the family. All used the label hyperactive to describe the girl. Ann and Paul existed in an enduring complementary relationship with outsiders, whom they saw as expert and knowledgeable, while they were "just parents."

Nearly all the activity with outsiders was carried on by Ann. She was the conduit between the family and larger systems. She took the child to doctors. She went to myriad school meetings and talked on the telephone to her daughter's teachers and school counselors. She would then translate these interactions to her husband, who remained distant from both Ann and the outside systems while encouraging her relationship to the doctors and teachers. Hence the outside systems unwittingly exacerbated an already troubled marital relationship by serving to relieve tensions between husband and wife in ways that prevented their ever needing to deal with issues of their own. As long as Paul supported his wife's interactions with outsiders, as long as Ann spent her major energies focused on systems outside her family, and as long as everyone's definition of the problem obviated change, the three systems were stabilized in ways that maintained the symptom and protected the marital relationship from any shift. The family's seating pattern at the first three sessions served as a metaphor for both intrafamily and intersystem relationships: Ann and Gina sat extremely close to each other and to the therapist, who potentially represented a new system entering the family's life, while Paul moved his chair into a far corner, away from his wife and the therapist but able to make frequent eye contact with his daughter.

Although the family had congenial relationships with medical and school people, their experiences with therapists had been threatening and dissatisfying. In the first session Paul told the therapist about a prior attempt at family therapy. The family dropped out after the second session when the previous therapist insisted that their marital relationship was the problem rather than Gina. The parents made it very clear that they were not coming to therapy for their marriage and that they got along fine. Further, the parents had a great deal of experience in taking their daughter to therapists for testing, play therapy, and behavior modification. In an offhand remark as he was leaving the first session, Paul muttered to himself, "I hope this isn't going to be like all those other times where the professionals ask all the questions, we answer, and then they keep findings to themselves." Paul resented the family's complementary relationship with helpers but seemed unable to shift to a different relationship.

Utilizing the father's remark at the end of the session as an important message, the therapy team decided that what was needed was to provide a different experience with helpers for the family in order to be effective. This unexpected experience would need to include affirming Paul as a full partner in any plans regarding Gina and shifting the complementary relationship between the family and outside systems to a symmetrical one. Moves internal to the family, requiring greater symmetry between the parents vis-à-vis their daughter, would be mirrored in the multisystem relationship.

The team's assessment was that for change to occur in the family's presenting problem, in the family's organization (which supported the symptom and was, in turn, maintained by the symptoms), and in the family's relationship to outsiders (which appeared both to be required by and to require the girl's problem), a major redefinition of the child's behavior was needed. The label "hyperactive" maintained all relationships as they have been described. A plan was developed that would require all three systems—family, medical, and school—to drop the label "hyperactive" and all the concomitant treatment. The team's point of view was that, if agreement were obtained that Gina was a normal girl who did some very naughty things, then all involved would be required to act differently toward her and toward each other. While this formulation sounds simple, it was in fact a bold notion, one that would require different responses from all the adults in the child's life. Further, the team recognized that the success of this plan hinged on orchestrating the cooperation of all three systems. If any one system refused the idea, the plan would be sabotaged and a fierce triangle would ensue, likely making matters worse.

The first step was to reframe the relationship of family, school, and physician as a partnership required to solve the problem. The message to the outside systems was that therapy could not be effective without their help—that the problem could not be solved without them. The expertise of each system was carefully delineated and affirmed. The therapy team was careful not to presume knowledge of medicine, education, or the family beyond its purview, but rather to seek guidance from each of these systems in such a way that put all three systems on the same level, thereby beginning to loosen the prior rigid complementarity between the family and outside systems. Competition among the larger systems was carefully avoided. Cooperation was deliberately sought.

The pediatrician was asked whether he would support a trial period without medication. He agreed that such a step was in order and that he would work with the family to accomplish this.

Having obtained the cooperation of the pediatrician, the therapy team worked to ready the family for the plan. Interventions were designed to move Paul a bit farther into the family sphere and to affirm both parents as experts on their own child, with knowledge of her that no professional possessed. Care was taken to confirm the years of effort put in by Ann on behalf of her child. This particular step was accomplished by a telephone call from the supervisor, behind the one-way mirror, to the mother. The effect of this was visible and dramatic, as Ann smiled and tears came to her eyes. Clearly, prior professionals working with the family had not taken time to let her know that her contributions were the sign of a loving and devoted mother. In the fourth session the parents entered and sat next to each other for the first time. They appeared more relaxed, and Ann turned to her husband for ideas.

The therapist decided to implement the plan. Gina was asked to leave the room, thus drawing a generational boundary. The therapist began by explaining to the parents the ways in which labels can shape and constrain behavior. He asked the parents if they would be willing to try a time-limited experiment. He carefully explained the team's point of view, which was that perhaps Gina was no longer hyperactive but a normal girl who engaged in very naughty behavior. He suggested that the only way to find this out would be for the parents to (1) tell her that she was no longer hyperactive and that they thought she was a normal girl who did naughty things, (2) stop the medication, (3) develop and implement a course of action with consequences that they both could support, and (4) work with the school to try the experiment there as well. The therapist asked the parents to talk this over with each other. The response was immediate approval of the plan, with Paul taking the lead and Ann agreeing. Without the therapist's prompting, Ann stated that they would need to contact the school and ask them to treat Gina as a normal girl, to expect her to do her work and cooperate, and to discipline her like any other child.

Gina came back into the session. The therapist asked the parents to tell her their decision. Both parents, starting with the father, informed her that they had decided tonight that she was no longer hyperactive, that she was a normal girl who did naughty things, and that when she misbehaved, she would be disciplined accordingly. The team noted that the parents dropped the term "experiment" in their explanation to the girl.

Any intervention provokes feedback within a system. The team's major concern was whether the family would verbally accept the intervention while disqualifying it at an analogic level. The following ensued: When Gina heard that she was no longer hyperactive but normal, she broke into a broad smile. The parents left the session arm in arm, and Paul waved to the team behind the mirror. The team understood that to be confirmation of the intervention.

On retrospective examination, the responses of all three systems to the change in labeling and the change in action required thereby may be seen in three stages, including an immediate period of euphoria, a homeostatic response, and a period of morphogenesis. Each period required an intervention planned by the therapeutic team. Involvement or contact with the medical and school systems was minimal during this period and occurred only at the direction of the family.

Immediately following removal of the hyperactive label, all three systems cooperated with the plan. The parents took Gina off medication and set clear rules for her. They reported that she began to follow their expectations and ceased to have tantrums at home. In subsequent weeks the physician kept an appropriate distance from the family, since the girl no longer had a medical problem. Paul attended a school meeting to instruct the school on implementing the plan, freeing Ann to engage in other activities. This was the family's decision, not directed by the therapist, and was the first time the father had gone to the school. School personnel who worked with Gina expected her to do her work and get along with other children. During the second week of the experiment Gina got into a fight at recess and was sent to the principal's office like any other child. No further incidents were reported.

When the family returned in 1 month reporting so much rapid change, the therapy team decided to predict dire consequences (Haley, 1976). The family was told that when change occurs so fast, it is not unusual for other difficulties to emerge. In particular, the therapist pointed out that Ann would be less occupied with doctors and school personnel and might become lonely. The intent of this comment was to continue loosening the bonds between the mother and outside systems. The therapist also hinted that many couples discover long-buried issues between themselves when a problem with a child no longer occupies their attention. The parents smiled at each other, and Paul remarked that the team just might be wrong this time.

The family was scheduled to be seen again a month later. Just prior to the session, Ann called. She was very upset and reported that Gina had become a problem again in school but not at home. She and her husband were frustrated. Ann was again more central and Paul more peripheral. The school was requesting that the family reinstitute the medication, and the parents were ready to reassume their one-down position with professionals. The team met and decided to see if the family was ready to close off the avenue of medication once and for all. The therapist called the family and instructed them to bring any remaining medication to the session. It was put to the parents that they must decide how they wanted the school to respond. The parents, in the presence of the girl, stated that they believed she did not need medication. The family members were given cards to read, entitled "Old Roles." These cards delineated the complementary roles in the family vis-à-vis hyperactivity. The family was invited to burn these cards, and Gina was given the matches to do so. The therapist then invited the family to bury the remaining medication and the ashes on a hill outside the clinic, while telling Gina that she was a normal girl. The somewhat bizarre nature of this ritual in a family that had relied on experts and on medication for 8 years seemed to function to free the family from its reliance on outsiders and to reaffirm its stance with the school just at a point when doubts on all sides were about to reestablish the original status quo.

At a 4-month follow-up, Gina was symptom free. When asked how Gina was doing, Ann remarked, "She's a normal 11-year-old, with a lot of energy!" Ann and Paul moved toward one another. Their previous united front had been dropped, and they were effectively negotiating conflicts with each other. The physician remained appropriately distant, seeing the family only when the child was physically sick. The school was treating her as they would any other child. Both parents kept in contact with the school as any parents would.

The therapy team decided to prescribe a planned relapse. They instructed the parents to ask Gina to pretend to have her old symptoms for 10 minutes once a week (Madanes, 1981). The response was immediate. Paul refused the intervention, stating that this was simply not necessary and that the team was wrong to suggest it. The team's understanding of Paul's response was that the work was done. Internally, the family had changed so that Gina's problems no longer functioned in her parents' marriage. By refusing the suggestion, the father was saying that the former implicit support for the girl's symptoms was no longer necessary or available. Externally, the family's relationship to outside systems was now symmetrical. By refusing the suggestion, the family was defining itself as the primary expert on its own life (Imber Coppersmith, 1982b).

This case exemplifies several elements involved in ongoing work with families and larger systems when labels are a key issue. Here the therapist took careful steps to secure the cooperation of the other larger systems involved and framed any success as contingent upon the work done by everyone. At no point were the other systems described negatively for their prior work. Rather the current work was framed as the next developmental step. Whenever possible, this approach, which positively connotes what has occurred, should be tried in order to minimize defensiveness, symmetrical escalation between therapist and larger systems, and the potential for triangulation. At each point in the case when action by the medical or school system was required, such action was carefully confirmed by the therapist. Whenever possible, the larger systems should be given credit for changes just as the family is given credit. This is especially important when the larger systems will remain in the family's life long after therapy is concluded, as is usually the case with medical and school systems.

In this case, the therapist was able to secure the cooperation of the other systems and was thus able to form a limited partnership with all of the involved systems. This position should be considered the first choice in ongoing work with a family and larger systems. Other choices will be delineated below.

Stigma

Families with a member who has been diagnosed as having a mental or physical illness or with a member involved with the criminal justice system often experience a sense of stigma from extended family, larger systems, and/or the wider community. Such stigma frequently exists in a long historical context regarding a given illness or condition. An example may be seen in long-standing attitudes towards the "mentally retarded." Such attitudes have historically included ostracizing the retarded person and his or her family, public policy that encouraged families to either reject or hide their retarded member, and the development of larger systems whose mandate was to keep the retarded out of any normal interaction with the wider community. While public policy has shifted to a focus on normalization and deinstitutionalization, in fact the stigmatizing process continues in many sectors of the wider community.

More recently, the disease of AIDS (Acquired Immune Deficiency Syndrome) has been met with a terrible stigmatizing process, one that extends to individuals in the so-called high-risk groups whether or not they have been diagnosed with the illness. This stigma is apparent at the level of larger systems, many of whom prefer not to treat AIDS patients.

While families may respond in many ways to stigma, what is important to consider is the effect of such stigma on individuals, on family relationships, on family–larger system interaction, and on a family's experience of itself in the wider community. Families may turn inward and cut off from larger systems whom they experience as hostile or pitying. They may become extremely combative with larger systems in defense of their ill member and of their integrity as a unit. Attributing these qualities to the family per se, without appreciating the effects of stigma, would be an error. Therapists entering such families must investigate the effect of stigma on family functioning and on family–larger system relationships. Usually the topic of stigma has not been discussed, but it should be discussed early. Often the therapist will need to adopt an advocacy stance, enabling the family to receive proper services. Initial work is best done at the family–larger system interface, since family therapy per se can easily contribute to a family's sense of stigma.

CASE EXAMPLE: A JOURNEY OUT OF HIDING

A single-parent family was referred for family therapy by a school system. The family consisted of Ms. Lane and her daughter, Samantha, 12. Samantha had been labeled mentally retarded shortly after her birth, and Mr. Lane left the family within a year of her birth. He maintained no contact and sent no support. Ms. Lane worked as a secretary. She supported herself and Samantha but had little time or money for socializing with other adults.

The referral for family therapy from the school stated that "Samantha was becoming increasingly unmanageable in the special classroom" and that Ms. Lane "needed parenting skills." Thus, blame for Samantha's behavior was located *in* the family by the school system.

Upon receiving the referral and before seeing the family, the therapist set out to find out a bit more about the referral. Samantha's school was a regular public school with separate classes for handicapped children. A visit to the school revealed that the "special" classrooms were hidden away in a far corner of the building. While other children went to the cafeteria for lunch, the handicapped children were required to eat lunch in their classrooms. The reason given for this was that "the normal children would make fun of them." The school did not see it as their responsibility to intervene in such attitudes and felt that they were protecting the handicapped children. No integrated classes were provided in any area.

The first session with Ms. Lane was spent discussing her experiences with larger systems in Samantha's behalf, focusing particularly on the present school. What emerged was a picture of stigma attached to Samantha's condition by a number of larger systems. Ms. Lane felt that her ex-husband also stigmatized Samantha, as did her extended family. Earlier in Samantha's life, Ms. Lane had tried to get her involved in Girl Scouts, but the troop leader complained that Samantha could not participate normally. In discussing her relationship with the school system, Ms. Lane stated that she felt that the principal and counselor seem to treat her as if she were retarded. (This experience has been described by many parents of handicapped children, in reference to their treatment by professionals involved with their child.)

During a discussion of how she understood the referral for family therapy, Ms. Lane said she was confused by it. She felt she was doing a good job parenting Samantha; however, she felt frustrated that she could not seem to get the school to respond to her requests to integrate

Samantha, at the very least for lunch and physical education. She also remarked that she felt isolated as the single parent of a child with handicaps. Over the years, she had given up socializing very much, because she felt most people were uncomfortable around Samantha. Thus the sense of stigma contributed to her growing isolation.

This discussion of Ms. Lane's experience with larger systems had never occurred before in all of her interactions with professionals on Samantha's behalf. Ms. Lane remarked that she often felt "dumped on" by helpers and that no one had ever bothered to elicit what it had been like for her to try to get services for Samantha.

Rather than embarking on family or individual therapy that would increase Ms. Lane's sense of being different and stigmatized, the therapist suggested a very different approach, one that would coach Ms. Lane in her dealing with the school system. The therapist and Ms. Lane became partners in Samantha's behalf, first assessing the unusual pattern that occurred between Ms. Lane and the school and then proceeding to develop strategies to get appropriate services for Samantha. The therapist spent some time teaching Ms. Lane about interacting with larger systems. Ms. Lane was unaware of her and Samantha's legal rights, and it was soon discovered that the school was violating the law regarding the education of handicapped children in the least restrictive environment. Ms. Lane was encouraged to meet with other parents of students in special education. Ms. Lane stated she had always felt too overwhelmed before to initiate such a meeting, but was ready to do so now. Such a meeting had not occurred before; it not only began to shift Ms. Lane's sense of isolation, it also began to develop a parent self-help group that took the issue of their children's education beyond the nonresponsive school personnel to the local board of education. Ms. Lane's sense of stigma was replaced by a sense of pride in her growing abilities to advocate for her daughter. She used the therapist as a coach but essentially accomplished what was required through the parent group. The school was required to implement new policies, and the handicapped children were appropriately integrated as required by law. Samantha's behavior at school began to improve as her mother grew in her sense of empowerment and as her treatment at the school changed.

Careful initial analysis of the referral was crucial in this case, in order to prevent the family therapist from becoming one more stigmatizing agent in the mother's life. The therapist engaged Ms. Lane in a way that respected her struggles, and conceptualized therapy as a coaching process at the family–larger system interface. Rather than functioning *for* Ms. Lane with the school, which would have continued her disempowerment, the therapist assisted her in developing a resource network with other parents, who together dealt with the school system. The positions of advocate, coach, and facilitator of natural resources are crucial elements when the therapist has assessed a macrosystem marked by stigma.

Secrecy

Labeling and stigma may combine in ways that produce secrets, both in families and between families and larger systems. For instance, the label "mental retardation" and the social stigma attached to this label resulted in many families hiding their mentally retarded member and producing a secret thereby. In turn, the treatment delivery for the mentally retarded, until the recent development of deinstitutionalization, hid the retarded from the community, thereby contributing to a pattern of secret keeping. In some larger systems, abusive treatment of the retarded formed yet another level of secrecy.

Homosexuality has been and in many quarters remains a secret both within families and between families and the outside world. The diagnostic label and subsequent stigma attached to certain physical illnesses have engendered patterns of secret keeping (e.g., cancer, AIDS) that operate at multiple levels of patient, family, larger system, and community. For example, a mother of a child with AIDS kept the diagnosis a secret from her other family members, fearing that they would ostracize her and the child when she most needed their support. The extreme stress of her child's illness was compounded by the stress of keeping the illness secret from family members, friends, and the school system, all of whom were told only that the girl had a severe kidney disease.

Secrecy has been examined primarily for its effects on internal family patterns and individual psychodynamics (Karpel, 1980; Paul & Bloom, 1970; Pincus & Dare, 1978.) The focus here is on the function and effects of secrets in the macrosystem.

Secrets between families and larger systems are metaphorical boundary markers. They may function to define alliances between those who know a particular secret. For example, a mother and a guidance counselor may have a secret that excludes a father, or a family may have a secret that is kept at all cost from outside systems. Relationships are defined and maintained by who knows the secret and who does not know it.

When one focuses less on the content of a secret and more on the pattern of secret keeping, an important phenomenon comes into view— the replication of secret-keeping behavior across the macrosystem. Thus, it is not unusual, when a larger system encounters a family whom they suspect is keeping a secret, for the larger system to begin to develop secrets from the family or from other larger systems involved in the case. Or representatives of one larger system may attempt to make secrets with representatives of another larger system, excluding the family or client. Soon the entire macrosystem is riddled with secrets and the concomitant distortion of communication, denial of perceptions, and avoidance of topics that might touch on the original secret, that one frequently encounters in patterns of secret keeping.

Larger systems may promote patterns of secret keeping by their approaches to particular problems or life-cycle issues. Such secrecy generally reflects wider social values and may shift as such values shift. For many decades, larger systems handling adoptions urged adoptive parents to keep their adopted child's status a secret. While such advice ultimately changed for families, the adoption system still maintains many dimensions of secrecy regarding biological parents. When social values and the larger system policies shaped by such values promote secrecy, people often experience a sense of shame regarding their circumstances (e.g., adoption, abortion, certain illnesses), and this sense of shame in turn promotes further secret keeping.

Larger systems often respond to a sense of secrets in families by pursuing the family for the content of the secret. Family members in turn may respond by distancing and setting up more rigid boundaries to the outside world. Escalating patterns of pursuit and distance, usually involving suspicion and blame, soon mark the macrosystem.

When secrets are maintained by labeling and stigma, then intervention often needs to occur on a broad community level. In the example of the secrecy that surrounded mental retardation, the process of deinstitutionalization that followed upon the opening of secrets regarding abusive treatment of many mentally handicapped people led to the abandonment of secret keeping at various levels of the macrosystem. Mentally handicapped people were no longer hidden away in institutions out in rural areas, but rather became visible members of communities. Families of the mentally handicapped no longer had to keep their status secret and thus remain isolated but could join with other families in self-help and handicapped-rights movements. The process of secret keeping could be reversed at multiple levels of the macrosystem.

CASE EXAMPLE: A 40-YEAR SECRET

A family was referred for family therapy by a psychiatric resident. The Johnson family consisted of two aging parents, Carrie and George, and two grown daughters, Catherine and Ellen, who had lived outside of the parents' home for many years. Carrie was referred for what was labeled a phobia, which included her refusal to touch anyone and a need to wash her hands very frequently. Her fears handicapped her in many ways, as she would not shop or travel. She spent most of her time at home and cried often. Carrie also talked about a fear of outsiders, who included everyone but her daughters. Helpers from larger systems were definitely in the category of outsiders.

The tone of the referral was one of intense frustration. Carrie had been hospitalized twice, and the larger psychiatric system had tried all manner of interventions with her, including medication, behavior modification, cognitive therapy, relaxation therapy, and a short course of marital therapy. The resident stated that he felt Carrie had some secret but that his attempts to uncover a secret had been rebuffed. He also reported a pattern of George and Carrie complaining to him privately about the other, but making him promise not to bring this up. Thus a pattern of secrecy between individual family members and outside helpers existed. Finally, secrecy existed within the larger psychiatric system, as Carrie was described privately as resistant, the family as uncooperative, and the case as hopeless. Such descriptions, clearly indicative of frustration and anger in the larger system, underpinned plans being discussed in the larger system, but not yet communicated to the family, to either send Carrie, who was in good health, to a nursing home or to recommend psychosurgery.

As family therapy began, the family presented a polite tone to the therapist. Exploration of patterns of conflict in the family were met with extreme denial that any conflict ever existed. Both daughters described keeping problems to themselves when they were growing up. Thus, secret keeping marked each member. Everyone insisted that all would be well in the family, if only Carrie's phobia could be solved.

A session was held with Catherine and Ellen, during which a pattern of secrecy emerged, similar to the one the resident described. Each parent would speak privately to a daughter, complaining about the other parent. When the daughter would attempt to raise this with both parents, the parents denied the conversation and feigned confusion. The daughters soon abandoned attempts to bring such issues into the open and instead spoke privately with each other, thus continuing a pattern of secrecy. Carrie's symptoms absorbed most of the family's attention and energy, diverting members from raising and resolving any other issues.

The family had a long history with larger systems, primarily psychiatric, regarding Carrie's problem. The major relationship pattern between Carrie and helpers was one of pursuit by the helpers and distance by Carrie. At various points, helpers would become frustrated and refer Carrie to someone else, and the pattern would begin again.

The sense of secrecy was palpable. Catherine and Ellen attempted to draw the family therapist into this pattern by urging her to see each parent separately. This request was declined, as it appeared isomorphic with existing family patterns and prior family–larger system patterns.

A very different plan was proposed. Catherine and Ellen were asked to keep a secret with the therapist, a metaphorical comment on secrets in the family. They were told that the therapy was stuck because the therapist was an outsider and that their help was needed in the next session as consultants to the therapist. They were asked if they would be willing to be behind the one-way mirror and from that position to assist the therapist. They were asked to keep this plan a secret from their parents, and they agreed.

When the family arrived for the session, the daughters were taken behind the mirror, shown how to operate the telephone, and asked to call the therapist anytime they felt that Carrie and George were being polite or diplomatic because the therapist was an outsider or anytime they felt new topics should be raised. Carrie and George were brought into the interviewing room, the plan for the session was explained to them, and they were given the opportunity to accept or decline the plan. As soon as they agreed, Ellen called to say she thought they were only agreeing out of politeness, and this message was relayed to the parents, who began to grapple with their daughters' perceptions. The entire session involved the therapist as a conduit from the daughters to the parents. Topics were raised regarding Carrie's and George's relationship, conflicts, and the pattern of each parent telling an issue to the daughters privately but denying it when they were together. Issues were raised involving the daughters' distress with ongoing family relationships that had previously been kept a secret between the daughters. Towards the end of the session, conflict emerged between the daughters, regarding whether it was a good idea to push the parents in this way. This conflict was reported to the parents, who were asked to go home and decide whether they felt it was a good idea to discuss issues openly and attempt to resolve them, or whether this might make things worse. The pattern of secret keeping was positively connoted as an act of protection among the members.

For 2 months, the therapist did not hear from Carrie and George. However, Catherine called and requested to see the therapist. In that session, she said that after the session in which the daughters served as consultants to the therapist, several issues emerged. The parents began to raise conflicts more openly, and Ellen revealed two secrets to the family, including her struggle with alcohol and that she and her boyfriend were living together and had been for 5 years, but had hidden this from the family. Catherine wanted to talk about an enormous and unexplained burden of guilt that she felt since childhood. The therapist began to work with her from a position of coach, regarding both her family of origin and her present family, as she had two grown sons who frequently took advantage of her. She also was concerned about a recent rise in her blood pressure and connected this to feeling a lot of family stress and being unable to deal with conflicts in her family.

After 2 months, Carrie and George returned to therapy and spontaneously began to speak about the history of their lives together. What emerged was a secret of 40 years' duration. Carrie had been pregnant with Catherine before she and George married. She was labeled as a bad girl by her family, and she and George were forced to move far away. The couple tried to keep Carrie's pregnancy a secret from George's family, who nonetheless found out and ostracized them. They decided then to keep the circumstances of Catherine's birth a secret from the children. This required keeping a lot of distance from their families and taking great care in any discussions, lest the topic touch on the family's origins. Communication in the family became more and more stilted and rigid. Distance and fear marked relationships. Interaction with larger systems was marked by this same fear and distance. Only Carrie's phobia, no doubt a metaphor for all of these family issues, kept family members talking to each other and to the outside world. George and Carrie never celebrated their anniversary or Catherine's birthday. Rituals that give a family a shared sense of itself were avoided and replaced by the rituals of Carrie's symptom.

This session broke the pattern of secrecy between the couple and the larger system. Carrie and George requested the therapist's assistance in telling the secret to their daughters. During this session, Catherine and Ellen told the parents that they had known this secret, or had at least suspected it, because of the ways in which the parents avoided anything to do with their wedding or anniversary. Carrie said she suspected they knew, because they never asked to see the couple's wedding pictures, even when others' wedding pictures were being seen. Thus an enormous knot of secret upon secret was unraveled, and the family's wall to the outside world came down. At the end of this session Carrie, who had not touched anyone in many years, took the therapist's hands in hers and thanked her.

Following the session in which the parents discussed their major secret with their daughters, Carrie requested a consultation with a medical person who could "teach her about germs." It is important to note that during one of her hospitalizations, Carrie had been forced to listen to a microbiologist on the topic of germs, but she simply dismissed his talk. Carrie's request to meet with a representative of a larger system, rather than her being *sent* to one, may be seen as a major shift in the family's relationship with larger systems. The family therapist facilitated this request. Following her meeting with the "germ expert," Carrie developed a plan of her own for overcoming her fears. She asked for and received a plan to end her dependency on antianxiety medication. She began to go out. She shopped and bought clothing for the first time in many years. She had her daughters and their families over for Easter dinner, which she had not done in several years. She began to play the piano again. When therapy ended, she brought the therapist a long-promised home-baked rhubarb pie (Imber-Black, 1986a).

For this family, social labeling (e.g., "illegitimate," "out of wedlock") combined with stigmatizing actions from families of origin and the community to result in a pattern of secret keeping, both in the family and between the family and the outside world. Larger systems encountering the family extended this pattern of secrecy in inadvertent and unplanned ways, thus contributing to rigidity in the macrosystem. The major intervention of placing the grown daughters behind the one-way mirror enabled several new relationship options. The larger system was now part of the family, rather than alien to it. The therapist was able to operate in a complementary one-down position, taking directions from the daughters, rather than in the previous and ineffective position of one-up, telling the family what it must do and encountering resistance, or the symmetrical position of keeping secrets from the family, just as the family kept secrets from the larger system. Family rules regarding secrecy were able to be broken in a nonjudgmental atmosphere. Asking family members to go behind the one-way mirror and to serve as consultants to the therapist is an intervention that has been used with repeated success when secrecy is an issue. In the case under discussion, the plan for such a session was also kept a secret, but in subsequent work with other families, utilizing the mirror and family members in this way, all members were told of the plan for the next session. At times, two or three sessions have been held, alternating who serves as consultant to the therapist. From behind the mirror, family members are able to comment with fewer constraints. Rules about secrecy can be circumvented. This intervention paradoxically utilized the boundary created by the mirror to generate greater openness. When a family has been involved with many larger systems, the position behind the mirror as consultant to the therapist is an empowering position. The family is able to be larger system to itself.

THERAPEUTIC POSITIONS

In cases involving ongoing work with families who are involved with larger systems, the therapist is required to have a wide repertoire of positions available. In family therapy, the concept of the position of the therapist has been a topic of much debate, as various models have insisted on particular appropriate positions for the therapist. Thus, proponents of the systemic model (Selvini Palazzoli et al., 1980a) have determined that neutrality is the only appropriate position for the therapist, while strategic and structural model theorists (Minuchin & Fishman, 1981; Fisch, Weakland, & Segal, 1982) have argued for a wider range of positions to insure therapist maneuverability. Bowenian therapists (Carter & McGoldrick Orfanidis, 1976) describe the therapist's position as that of coach, combining avoidance of unplanned side-taking with very planful teaching and directives.

For the therapist working with families and larger systems, careful initial assessment of the family's usual relationship with helpers will often guide the therapist regarding the issue of position, enabling the family to experience a different relationship and hence a different macrosystem than that which has been maintaining problems. Since most families who have problematic relationships with larger systems tend to experience disempowerment, it is crucial that whatever positions the therapist takes in the ongoing conduct of the work, the ultimate outcome should be an empowered position for the family. This movement from disempowerment to empowerment is reflected in the three cases discussed above, which included a wide range of positions for the therapist.

Positions to consider when working with families and larger systems include neutrality, complementarity, negotiator, coach and advocate, and partnership.

1. When one first encounters a family that is involved with larger systems, the most useful position to adopt is one of neutrality, since this will enable a careful assessment of the macrosystem without prematurely taking sides in a way that would limit later effectiveness. Such neutrality does not imply coldness or distance, but rather a nonpartial information-gathering stance. Often such use of neutrality provides a new experience to the family and to the representatives of larger systems, since public-sector macrosystems are frequently marked by secret alliances and by blame. Since the neutral stance is ultimately disinterested in the issue of family empowerment vis-à-vis larger systems, it is limited as a therapeutic position for ongoing work, especially when the family is being stressed or disempowered by the larger system.

2. Families who are in ongoing relationships with larger systems frequently have become used to an enduring one-down complementary position in which they are the recipients of care, advice, direction, and criticism from helpers who occupy the one-up complementary position. Families may seek to solve this problem in unusual ways, as did the couple described in "A family taking care of its helpers," in Chapter 4, who behaved in protective ways towards a bevy of helpers, thus placing themselves in the one-up position. Other families may find themselves in an escalating complementary cycle whereby more and more help results in more and more helplessness. Here the therapist may wish to deliberately adopt a one-down complementary position, introducing an unusual relationship with a helper. Such complementarity may be achieved in a number of ways, including seeking the family's advice, utilizing family members as consultants as in the case "A 40-year secret" discussed above,

or purposefully fashioning interventions that put the family in charge of the issue of help.

3. In the negotiator conduit position, the therapist stands *between* the family and larger systems, serving as mediator, translator, and shuttle diplomat. This position is particularly useful when anger is high between the family and larger systems. To be effective in this position, the therapist must have credibility with both the family and the larger systems. The work involved is similar to negotiation, in which each side is asked to make certain moves and concessions in order to achieve resolution. Skills of reframing and conflict resolution are heavily utilized.

4. One adopts a coaching and advocacy position with the family vis-à-vis larger systems when it has been determined that the larger system is unlikely to move and clients' rights are being violated. The case "A journey out of hiding" described above is an example of such work. The therapist teaches about family–larger system relationships, guides the clients in determining rights (for instance, educational rights for handicapped children), advocates for the clients in the larger systems, and coaches the clients to advocate for themselves and their families. The therapist discusses strategies with the client and may utilize role-playing and rehearsals. The therapist positions himself or herself frankly on the family's side in ways that are definitely nonneutral. Such coaching and advocacy is enhanced by the therapist's familiarity with a systemic paradigm that enables the development of interventions sensitive to reciprocal responses and that facilitates deescalation of conflict and blame.

5. A partnership position is useful when cooperation has been facilitated in the macrosystem, and ongoing work between the family and larger systems is required. In the case "From 'hyperactive' to 'normal but naughty'" described above, such a partnership was developed among the family, the school, the physician, and the therapist. Movement towards such partnerships is facilitated by the therapist's taking a stance that affirms the unique contributions of each system to the resolution of a problem. This stance minimizes competition and carefully delineates the different areas of expertise available. The family is connoted as on the same level as representatives of the larger systems, and the therapist takes care to draw forth the family's areas of expertise regarding its own members.

During work with any one case, a therapist may shift among the various positions described above. The work is active and planful, and the therapist should be cognizant of his or her position and intentions in adopting a particular position. Ongoing work with a family involved with larger systems should result both in problem resolution and in a family that is more empowered to make its way in the macrosystem.

CHAPTER 7

Women, Families, and Larger Systems

Large human service delivery systems at once reflect and are shaped by sociopolitical forces and ideological beliefs of the wider culture. Larger systems stand between the family and the wider social context and generally represent long-standing beliefs extant in the society, including unquestioned beliefs and stereotypes regarding women's roles. The process of change in the culture at large tends to reach the larger systems slowly, often creating a lag time, wherein the larger systems continue to reflect old agendas in their interactions with families. Much of our current human service delivery network has roots in the post–World War II period, a time that glorified the nuclear family, focused on family togetherness, and defined variant family forms as aberrant. While the modern women's movement has radically altered options for women and available family forms, the larger systems delivering services to families most often continue to operate out of old and unexamined norms that support traditional family organizations (e.g., two parents) and traditional family functioning (e.g., father working outside the home, mother working inside the home). The feminist critique and challenge has been essentially ignored by large public-sector systems such as welfare, public schools, and hospitals, resulting in a pattern of service delivery that reinforces stereotyped views of families and women's places in those families.

Many larger systems lack a perspective that affirms the historical, political, social, and economic context within which their work exists. It is this context that continues to support traditional sex roles, financial disparity between men and women, the mythical autonomous nuclear family, and the value of productivity over relationship. Without an appreciation of this context, the larger systems are able to remain blind to the effects of policies and procedures that support an agenda that blames women for the problems in their families.

184

BRIEF EXAMPLE: AN "OVERINVOLVED" MOTHER

A family was referred for family therapy by a public school system. The family consisted of two parents and a 10-year-old son, Shawn. Shawn had severe learning disabilities and frequently had trouble getting along at school, because other children would tease him. The referral for family therapy was requested because the school felt that Shawn's mother was overinvolved and handicapping Shawn's progress.

Before accepting the referral, the therapist went to the school to speak to school personnel involved with Shawn's program. Each spoke of the overinvolvement of Shawn's mother, citing her frequent telephone calls to discern how Shawn was doing and her anxiety about other children harming Shawn. The guidance counselor stated, "Poor Shawn— he can't get out from under Mother's thumb!"

The therapist inquired about the school's pattern of contact with the family. All appointments to discuss Shawn were made with the mother at a time when the father could not be available. No one had met Shawn's father or talked to him by telephone. Recently the school had been giving less information to Shawn's mother, stating that she was making Shawn anxious. Receiving less information, Shawn's mother had been calling the school more often. Thus a fairly classic distance–pursuit cycle was under way. The school also affirmed that Shawn's learning problems were quite severe and that he would be handicapped in educational and vocational pursuits.

Rather than beginning family therapy by accepting a referral that blamed the mother, the therapist suggested a session at the school involving both parents and the school personnel. At that session, care was taken to delineate the mother's expert knowledge of her son, knowledge which the school had ignored. It became apparent at the meeting that the father had delegated all responsibility for Shawn to his wife but frequently criticized her overinvolvement in a pattern similar to the school's. Instead of initiating family therapy, the therapist suggested a series of meetings between the school and the parents, suggesting that while it was important that Shawn's father attend these meetings, it was equally important that Shawn's mother be considered a "member of Shawn's educational team." The direction of the work included reframing the problem from one of overinvolved mother to one of need for communication between home and school, engaging the father *without* suggesting that the mother should disengage, and affirming the mother's special knowledge of her son as a resource for the school to utilize, rather than disqualify. As the mother was affirmed in her role on behalf of her son, her anxious presentation to the school lessened. With several people now on his side and the conflict between his mother and the school dissipated, Shawn, while still severely handicapped, began to function much better in the school setting.

ISSUES BETWEEN LARGER SYSTEMS AND WOMEN

When one examines the relationship between larger systems and women clients, several salient issues emerge.

The tendency to view problems in the family as either the woman's fault or her responsibility to solve. Many larger systems tend to engage a woman in a treatment process and orient all change-related activities and responsibilities around her, even when the identified problem may be a handicapped child, an alcoholic husband, or a rebellious adolescent. This tendency is especially marked in medical and educational systems. The nature of this phenomenon, by which larger systems designate women as the client, is illustrated in a National Academy of Sciences report on bereavement (*New York Times*, September 22, 1984) that said that "grief counseling was not for everyone but might be particularly helpful for some *widows* and for *mothers* who lose newborn babies" (emphasis added). What is especially curious is that this conclusion follows upon data that cites the dangers for both men and women following close personal loss, yet it is women who are seen as the necessary consumers of the assistance offered by larger helping systems.

BRIEF EXAMPLE: A LARGER SYSTEM BLAMES A WOMAN

A couple, Mr. and Mrs. Leon, in their mid-30s, were referred for a consultation. The couple had three young children. Mr. Leon had chronic migraine headaches since young adulthood. He had coped with the headaches until 2 years ago, when they worsened and he began several stays in the hospital. Recently he lost his job, and Mrs. Leon began to work outside the home for a minimum wage. The consultation was requested by the hospital because all medical efforts were failing, a psychiatric hypothesis was being considered, since Mr. Leon was extremely depressed, and hospital personnel were in great conflict with Mrs. Leon.

What emerged during the interview were the disparate beliefs that Mr. and Mrs. Leon held towards traditional health care. Mr. Leon stated that he had absolute faith in modern medicine and that he was certain that in time the hospital would help him. Mrs. Leon believed in holistic healing and felt betrayed by what she saw as her husband's alliance with medical personnel, who in fact were not helping him. She felt he was a "guinea pig" and was extremely angry with him for allowing this and with the hospital for continuing to treat him, despite repeated failures. She recounted several angry interactions between herself and hospital personnel, which she believed were the result of her refusal to agree with their treatment plans. Over time, her husband's physicians told her less and less regarding their decisions. The personnel in the hospital stipulated that she was a "kooky woman," and some felt that the exacerbation of Mr. Leon's headaches were her fault. Mrs. Leon's refusal to accept a complementary relationship with the health care system, in which they made decisions and she went along, a relationship that mirrors traditional male–female roles in the culture, seemed especially to draw forth the ire of the hospital personnel.

As seen in the example above, the tendency to view family problems as belonging to the woman often unwittingly allies larger systems with people and patterns, in the family and in the culture at large, that are always defining the problem in this way. It is not unusual to see a peripheral or disengaged father hand his overinvolved wife over to helpers to calm her down. Without examination of the larger systems' place as both the carrier of cultural messages about women and the ally of family members, a woman- and mother-blaming stance becomes common.

The disqualification of women's concerns and experiences by the larger systems. The term "overinvolved mother" is frequently used by larger systems to describe women whose children are experiencing difficulties. Inherent in the term is both criticism of the mother and implicit blame for her child's problem. This label neatly ignores the sociohistorical development of North American families, which placed women at home, caring for children. It also ignores the often profound requirement in families with ill or handicapped children, or in poor families living in unsafe neighborhoods, for mothers to be vigilantly involved on behalf of their child's safety and well-being. Women who are not so vigilant may find that they are labeled by the larger systems as neglectful.

Women's relationships with other women relatives and friends are often designated as overly close or symbiotic. The particular importance of such relationships to the family organization of poor and minority families is often ignored by larger systems. Thus, a single black mother who lives with her own mother may be called into a school or clinic about a child, while the grandmother's crucial presence in the system is either ignored or actively undermined.

BRIEF EXAMPLE: IGNORING A GRANDMOTHER

A poor young mother, seemingly a single parent, came to a pediatric clinic with her 5-year-old daughter. While there, she complained about her child's behavior and asked the pediatrician for his advice. In subsequent appointments, it became clear that she was unable to follow his advice because it differed markedly from her mother's advice. She lived with her mother, and so her household actually contained two adult women who served as parents to the little girl. Rather than assume that the grandmother was an important resource in this family, whose ideas he needed to understand and utilize, the pediatrician began to push the young mother harder to follow his advice. He never contacted the grand-mother. The case culminated in a referral for therapy for the mother, because the pediatrician thought she was becoming depressed. The referral note stated that this was a "single-parent family, lacking a male role model." The pediatrician clearly assumed that a female-headed family was deficient, made no effort to enhance existing strengths in the two women, and seemed to believe that two women only equaled a single parent.

The communication of mixed and binding messages to women from representatives of larger systems. Since the culture at large frequently communicates mixed messages to women, it should not be surprising to find similar communication from larger systems to women clients. Thus, at one and the same time, women are counted on by larger systems to be the emotional repository for their families and are designated overemotional and unable to cope. Women are given the responsibility for handling issues of distress in family members and are simultaneously criticized for initiating and maintaining patterns of enmeshment. Mothers are often contacted and engaged by larger systems and referred to multiple helpers via a referral system that highlights deficits rather than strengths and identifies specific helpers for every problem. If a mother cooperates with this pattern of referral, she easily becomes the conduit of information from the larger systems to the rest of the family and may find that her centralized position leads her to be designated as overinvolved. If the mother refuses to enter relationships with myriad larger systems, she will frequently be designated as resistant and uncooperative or told that she is not doing all that she can do for her child.

In a wider culture that places a premium on independence and eschews outside help, women are often cajoled to utilize helpers or are required by the exigencies of social policy to be dependent on larger systems (e.g., welfare). While the woman's dependency is thus fostered, she is simultaneously encouraged to accept solutions to children's problems that stress autonomy to the exclusion of interdependence, especially for male children. Women are thus invited to be inappropriate role models for their children.

BRIEF EXAMPLE: DENIGRATING THE MOTHER–SON SUPPORT SYSTEM

A family consisting of a mother, a stepfather, and an 11-year-old boy was referred for a consultation by a group home where the boy was residing.

While the boy's conflictual relationship with his stepfather was given as a cause for concern, staff were much more concerned over what they deemed as "overcloseness and overinvolvement" of the mother with her son. During the consultation, a picture emerged of mother and son living together since the boy was 6 months old, when his father left, until the stepfather entered when the boy was 9. Mother and son lived far away from other relatives and were an important source of support to each other. Adjustment to the entry of the stepfather was difficult for all concerned. When the boy began to misbehave, the mother took him to a counselor, who told her that she was too close to him and that it was crucial for his development that she distance. The mother wanted very much to be a good mother, and so she followed the advice of the professional, who she thought knew better than she did. As she distanced, her son's behavior became worse. She was counseled to distance more. The boy became very depressed, culminating in his placement in the group home.

By the time of the consultation, the mother was also very depressed and confused over whether to get close to her son or not. Clearly, the message she had received from the larger system was that she was somehow toxic to her son. Her moves to distance from him, as advised, were experienced by him as losing her, and he blamed his stepfather. The larger system's inability to preserve the strengths inherent in this mother–son dyad, while assisting in the shifts necessitated by the new stepfamily organization, contributed to the deterioration of both mother and son.

Special triangles involving women clients. Triangles involving two or more larger systems and women clients often operate in ways that infantilize the woman as the larger systems argue over who knows best for the woman. The possibility that the woman might know what's best for herself or might be an equally contributing member to an evolving consensus is generally ignored. Since wars between helpers usually contribute to a client's confusion and erode confidence, the triangle easily becomes self-perpetuating.

Such triangles may also emerge between more traditional larger systems involved with a woman client and newer systems whose avowed purpose is to advocate for women's concerns (e.g., shelters, sexual abuse programs, etc.) but who may perform such advocacy without a sense of systemic analysis to guide their work.

Interaction between larger systems and female-headed single-parent families. The relationship between larger systems and female-headed single-parent families is often marked by an interaction of similar beliefs about single-parent families, designating such families as inherently lacking. This similarity of beliefs easily facilitates a pattern in which the single parent relies on adults from larger systems to become the missing parent, and helpers erroneously believe that it is their role to do so. Strengths inherent in the single-parent family form are not validated by the larger systems. Work to enhance existing competencies in the single-parent mother is eschewed. Morawetz and Walker (1984) describe the relationship between single-parent mothers and representatives of larger systems as one where mothers often receive the message that professionals can make children behave well but the mother is incapable of doing so. Here children easily get involved in triangles between their own mothers and outside helpers, since to improve with such outside help that disqualifies the mother is to be disloyal to her, while to remain symptomatic continues the criticism of the mother from the outside systems.

BRIEF EXAMPLE: WHO HOLDS THE COOKIE JAR LID?

A single-parent mother of three teenage girls was referred for family therapy by her welfare worker, who cited the "chaotic household." The welfare worker had made many referrals of the family to therapy before. Each ended with the therapist stating that the mother had grown too dependent on therapy. In a discussion with the mother about the prior therapies, she stated that she did not feel the other therapists had really understood how her family worked and that each had unilaterally ended the therapy.

In the new therapy the therapist, who was a male trainee, began by trying to understand what the mother meant about how her family worked. The family was organized as four women living together. The mother stated that, as her girls got older, it simply made more sense to try to live together this way. The welfare worker's stipulation that the family was chaotic seemed to refer to this lack of hierarchy in their living arrangement. This way of being together worked much of the time, but when there were disputes, the mother tried to assert her authority, the girls would not pay attention to her, the mother would complain to her welfare worker, and a referral would be made to a therapist who would try to impose hierarchy in the family.

Rather than repeat these prior unsuccessful attempts, the therapist initiated a series of sessions that affirmed this less hierarchical arrangement, and posed questions to settle the issue of what to do when there were disputes. Therapy began by asking the family to look closely at what was working in their arrangement and then moved to what needed to change. The pattern of the larger system criticizing the mother was eschewed. All three girls agreed that they thought their mother should have the final word but stated that they had not felt listened to in the prior therapies. One daughter stated that in a prior therapy, the therapist kept saying to the mother, "You have to be in charge!" without delineating the occasions or the methodology. During the course of the therapy several different issues, such as curfew, school attendance, and smoking, were raised and successfully negotiated.

It became evident to the therapist that the time to end therapy had arrived, but he wanted to be careful to not repeat the prior endings that had left the mother out of the decision. He raised his point of view and then elicited the mother's. She stated that she believed things were going well *because* they were in therapy. She said to the therapist, "It is as if we are all in a cookie jar, and you have your hand on the lid to the cookie jar. When we come here every week, you are able to carefully take the lid off the cookie jar and we can talk. We still run into some trouble at home." Thus, credit for things going well was being placed in the therapist's hands. The mother's own sense of empowerment was not quite there. This was the same point reached in other therapies when the mother had been stipulated as too dependent on therapy. One may hypothesize that this was the only way the mother knew that therapy ended.

The therapist chose a very different direction, avoiding the prior treatment failures. Again affirming the family's more collaborative style, he asked them to all go shopping for "just the right cookie jar." When they had found it, they were to meet at home the following week during the time when they ordinarily came to therapy. The mother was asked to start a meeting with "her hand on the lid of the cookie jar." She could then pass the lid to others who wished to speak. The following week they were to bring the cookie jar to their regular therapy appointment. When they showed up for the appointment, the mother did not wait for the therapist to begin the session. Rather, she started with her hand on the lid of the cookie jar and passed it to him when she had finished describing their very successful meeting the week before. The therapist again asked her about therapy. She replied that she would like to do 3 weeks of meeting at home and then come in to see him. Therapy tapered off in 2 months, rather than ending abruptly as in the past. The passing of the cookie jar lid, initiated at each meeting by the mother, came to symbolize a family style that was both collaborative and hierarchical when necessary. The mother's sense of empowerment vis-à-vis her family *and* larger systems grew. When therapy ended, she brought the therapist a second cookie jar to keep for other families who might need it.

The cultural belief that children require male role models in order to develop adequately is frequently invoked by helpers working with single-parent mothers, to the exclusion of strengths that the mother herself may exhibit. Such mothers are often told that they must engage with male helpers for their children. Big Brothers are often recommended before the helpers have investigated to find out if male relatives, such as uncles or grandfathers, or reliable male friends of the family are available. Interventions to reconnect the single-parent family to natural supports are often not investigated or fully facilitated. The competencies of single-parent women are particularly ignored in referrals for Big Sisters.

CASE EXAMPLE: A THIRD OPINION

A consultation was sought by a family therapist who was working with low socioeconomic class families within a large, multidisciplinary, multimodality program. Due to the nature of this single larger system, families were often engaged with multiple helpers within the one institution. Other professional and paraprofessional community resources were also utilized.

The family brought for consultation was a single-parent family, consisting of Ms. Montero and her two children, Ida, 11, and Joseph, 8, who was the identified patient (see Figure 7-1).

The family had been a single-parent family since shortly after Joseph's birth. Joseph showed some congenital problems that affected his development, and Mr. Montero left at this time. Early in the separation, the father had threatened to take the children and leave the country. At that time Ms. Montero sought and received an order that allowed only supervised visitation between father and children, which Mr. Montero declined to exercise. The family and Mr. Montero were thus cut off. In presenting the case for consultation, the therapist noted that the subject of the children's father never came up in therapy, and while a lot was known to the therapist about Ms. Montero's extended family, nothing was known about Mr. Montero's extended family. It is important to note that both the therapist and his supervisor were male, entering a family in which a father was proclaimed to be "missing" and the identified patient was an "angry son." The stage was readily set for a therapy that focused on issues of Joseph's "need for a man," rather than on his need for a strong and competent mother.

Ms. Montero's extended family consisted of two sisters and a mother, as her father had died shortly after Joseph's birth. After the separation, Ms. Montero and her children moved in with the next oldest sister, Alice, where they lived until 1 year ago, at which time they moved to a place of their own. While complaints about Joseph's anger had been going on since his toddlerhood, everyone agreed that the situation had worsened when the family moved into their own place. The belief easily arose in the extended family that Ms. Montero could not manage her family on her own, and she was the object of much advice. No one conceptualized the move per se as a transition to actual single-parenthood, an equally plausible explanation for Joseph's escalation.

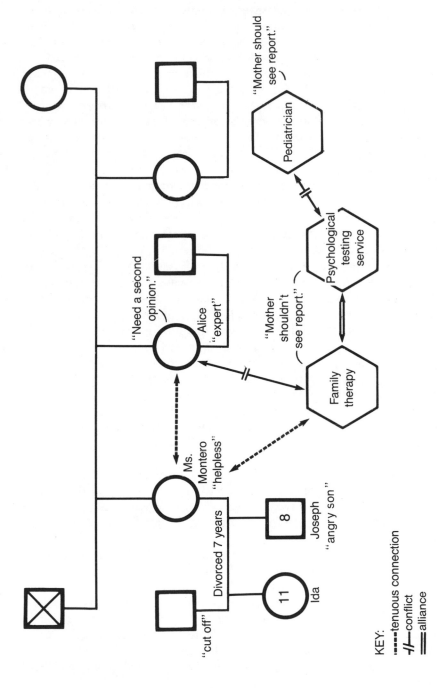

KEY:

▪▪▪▪ tenuous connection
━╫━ conflict
═══ alliance

Figure 7-1. Single-parent family, extended family, and larger–systems conflicts.

193

Ms. Montero's youngest sister, Tammy, was Joseph's godmother and felt particularly inclined to correct Ms. Montero and advise her regarding the raising of Joseph. She was also the only member of the extended family to have finished college, and so the family tended to accept her point of view as more valid, more professional.

When Joseph's behavior at home towards his mother and sister became increasingly untenable, including long-lasting tantrums and hitting them, Ms. Montero sought the advice of her pediatrician, who referred the family for therapy. This was about 1 year before the consultation. At the time, shortly after the move, Ms. Montero was making other changes in her life, including going to work outside the home and going to college part-time. In short, her own competencies as a woman and as a single parent were rising, but Joseph's behavior and family members' responses to it made her doubt herself. Messages from family members and others questioning her working and going to school contributed to her uncertainties.

The therapy had focused primarily on Joseph. During the year of therapy, in which little progress appeared to have been made, a number of working methods were attempted, including a lot of advice to Ms. Montero on parenting, getting Joseph a Big Brother, and finally sending Joseph for psychological testing. It was this final intervention that had provoked a crisis for which the consultation was sought.

The psychological testing had been done about 2 months before the consultation, and the written report had been extremely negative, pessimistic, and frightening, suggesting that Joseph would likely end up in residential treatment. In a paternalistic way, the actual report had not been shown to Ms. Montero by the tester, who instead simply talked with her, believing she "could not handle seeing the report." Various members of the larger system agreed that she should not see the actual report, feeling it would be too upsetting. The point of view towards Ms. Montero was that she was not competent to receive a written copy of the report and know how to make sense of it. Ms. Montero's pediatrician, adopting a different point of view towards her rights and competencies as a parent, showed her the report.

At this juncture, Tammy became more involved and insisted on coming to a therapy session to find out more about this report. She appeared very angry towards the therapist and questioned his competence to deal with Joseph, since the report said Joseph was so disturbed. She insisted that Ms. Montero seek a second opinion and said she would arrange for this at another hospital. Thus Ms. Montero, as a single parent striving to be competent with her children, found herself in a triangle of massive proportions between her extended family and her therapist.

At the consultation, both children were well behaved, and Ms.

Montero reported that both did extremely well in school. She then began to report that Joseph's behavior at home had begun to improve in the last 6 weeks. She had no explanation for this but felt that she was having an easier time being firm with him and settling him down if he did begin to get angry. Joseph, who had been quite isolated, had also begun to make friends. In short, something significant was changing in the family.

Ms. Montero then began to describe difficulties with her extended family and the demand that she get a second opinion. She disagreed with much of the report about Joseph but didn't really see the need for more testing. However, she felt she could not stand up to her sister and described that her own role in the family was that of peacekeeper. In response to questions about bringing extended family members to therapy, she stated strongly that she was against this, as she wanted more privacy for her nuclear family, which she felt she had never had. In her own words, she was making a plea for clearer boundaries and expressing the wish that the therapy would coach her to accomplish this.

She also expressed confusion about the therapy and the report. Since the report had been so dire regarding Joseph, she could not understand why therapy was meeting only once every 3 weeks. She was clearly thoughtful and deliberate regarding her children and her family.

She stated that Joseph was seeing a Big Brother and that he also did many things with his two uncles. The natural resource of the uncles had never been discussed in therapy.

The consultation focused briefly on the children's father. Ms. Montero was obviously extremely angry with him. No one discussed him at home or in therapy. The children insisted that they were not interested in him and did not think about him. Of note was the fact that he regularly paid child support through the welfare office and was clearly still present in the system in many ways. Rather than lecture Ms. Montero about his importance, which would simply replicate the pattern of advice giving from professionals and extended family on myriad other topics, the consultant chose to plant seeds by raising questions about the father's possible involvement with the children at a later time, suggesting that as adolescents it would not be unusual for the children to seek contact with their father.

The end-of-session intervention sought to empower Ms. Montero as the head of her family and to reconceptualize treatment as a coaching partnership. The consultant began by framing Ms. Montero as the expert on her children, the one who knew them better than anyone. Her competencies as a single parent were stressed, and the family's single-parent status was dated from their move into their own home a year earlier. The escalation of Joseph's angry behavior was normalized and connected to this transition in both the nuclear and extended family. The report on Joseph was framed as one opinion, rather than truth, as evidenced by the obvious progress in Joseph's behavior in the last little while. Since Ms. Montero had indicated that she felt bound to seek the second opinion that her sister wanted, this too was highlighted as an *opinion*. Ms. Montero was then asked if she would be willing to construct a report about Joseph, about Ida, about their relationship as brother and sister, about their relationship to her as mother and head of the family, about present issues in the family, and about her preferred future for her family. This report was labeled a "third opinion" and placed at a metalevel to the other two reports.

Ms. Montero was then asked to determine with the therapist how often therapy should occur, and therapy was reframed as a partnership that would include coaching Ms. Montero about relationships with her family of origin.

Several of the issues between women and larger systems discussed above were present in this case. The complementary relationship between single parents and professional helpers was evident, complicated by a triangle between family, extended family, and larger systems. The consultation elicited and intervened in a pattern between Ms. Montero and her extended family, a pattern replicated by the relationship with professional helpers who continually defined Ms. Montero as one-down, disempowering her as a mother and head of her own family. The consulting interview deliberately focused on her strengths, rather than on deficits. Advice giving was eschewed in favor of a process of coaching, in which Ms. Montero would give a lot of input, determine directions, and use professionals as resources, rather than as those who knew better than she did. Inviting her to construct a report, whose validity was equal to any professional report written and which would serve as a guide for any subsequent therapy, affirmed and empowered her position in the macrosystem.

WOMEN'S ROLES IN LARGER SYSTEMS

Women are not only family members and the clients of larger systems, they are also often workers within larger systems. As family therapists increasingly add consultation to larger systems to their repertoire of systemic assessment and intervention, it is crucial to attend to the issue of gender as it plays out in the larger systems seeking such consultation.

The consultant may be confronted with a variety of configurations. The first involves consulting to systems in which there are traditionally female subsystems within larger, male-dominated systems. Examples include health care systems, in which nurses form the predominantly female and subordinate subsystem, and educational systems, where women are most often in the position of teachers, while men generally fill the administrative positions. As women's roles change in work systems, these generalizations will begin to shift, but they remain salient currently. These larger systems replicate traditional male–female roles in the wider culture. A serious gender issue for the consultant entering such systems is the frequent disqualification of women's complaints within the larger system. Problems beginning in the largely women's subsystem of the larger system are often ignored until they reach epic proportions and may be less amenable to intervention.

The second issue involves the emergence of women's leadership in systems that previously did not have women occupying leadership positions. Often such women are in a very difficult bind. If they behave authoritatively and hierarchically, as they have seen male leaders do, they may find themselves criticized as "bitches"; if they behave collaboratively, with an emphasis on preserving relationships, they may be criticized for being too soft, too feminine.

The larger systems seldom acknowledge gender as one of the key issues in problems or the preferred solutions. A consultant who attends to this issue is able to reframe struggles by making the gender issue more visible.

BRIEF EXAMPLE: MAKING GENDER VISIBLE

A public high school sought a consultation for what were termed "degenerating relationships" in the guidance office. A new head of guidance, Ms. Kraus, had been hired 1 year previously. She replaced another woman, Ms. Appel, who had voluntarily stepped down due to illness in her family but who maintained a position within the department. Ms. Appel's leadership style had been highly collaborative. However, she was criticized for this by the central administration, who felt she was not tough enough. In seeking her replacement, the administration deliberately sought what they referred to as a "stronger" person. The guidance staff consisted of six professional counselors and three secretaries, all women. The central administration consisted of a superintendent, an assistant superintendent, a principal, and two assistant principals. All were men.

When Ms. Kraus entered the system, she was instructed by the administration to be tough. Unfortunately, she interpreted this message to mean that she should not join with Ms. Appel, who offered to introduce her to the system, which offer Ms. Kraus declined. In a short time, rumblings of dissatisfaction with Ms. Kraus's leadership began to be heard from the staff. These were ignored by the administration and disqualified as "women's jealousies." Complaints that, had they come from a staff of men, would likely have been taken very seriously were simply discounted. The situation deteriorated, and as staff morale plummeted, absenteeism grew.

The situation had reached crisis proportions before consultation was sought. While there was a variety of ways to conceptualize issues, the consultant chose to examine the system from a gender perspective, looking closely at the phenomenon of women turning against each other in a male-run larger system. The values of leadership that Ms. Kraus had adopted were those that seemingly would ally her with the administration but that had in fact alienated her from her staff and made successful work impossible. As the consultant raised issues of leadership style with Ms. Kraus, it became clear that she felt bound by the mandate to be tough issued to her by the administration, while at the same time not feeling comfortable with executing this style. Consequently, she tried even harder to be tough, assuming that she would be judged on her capacity to do so. Ironically, by the time of the consultation, not only the guidance staff was blaming her, but also the administration was. She found herself scapegoated and confused that the administration was blaming her for doing the very thing it had initially asked her to do.

The consultant raised gender issues as an important dimension of what was occurring. At first, this conceptualization was dismissed by the participants, who continued to blame Ms. Kraus. Ms. Kraus, however, quickly began to see the bind she was in and started to shift her behavior towards other guidance staff in ways that fit with a leadership style she preferred. She began to seek more input from her staff. As she did so, they began to cooperate with her more. She remarked that she realized that strong leadership did not mean autocratic leadership. The consultant also worked with the administration, highlighting the need to take complaints seriously much earlier. Questions were posed that raised the different treatment of men's and women's subsystems within the larger system. In short, the consultation turned on a consciousness-raising effort done in a way that highlighted the larger system's embeddedness in the wider culture, rather than blaming individuals. This approach enabled an examination of sexism within the institution and the implementation of school-wide workshops on sexism. These discussions, in turn, led to the beginnings of curriculum development on gender issues.

While this consultation certainly did not alter the attitudes of all of the participants, it did provide an opening for the examination of the institution's gender issues and sexism, which had remained invisible prior to the consultation. Through noticing and highlighting gender issues, the consultant was able to intervene in an escalating scapegoating process that would have soon culminated in the extrusion of Ms. Kraus and no real change in the larger system.

CONCLUSION

The family therapist working with women, their families, and larger systems requires special cognizance of the unspoken and unquestioned assumptions that underpin the work of most larger systems regarding women.

Simplistic hypotheses that covertly or overtly blame women for their circumstances must be challenged. Formulations that link symptoms only to individuals and families, while ignoring historical, social, political, and economic constraints that have shaped and determined women's positions in families, require reworking. Sensitivity to actual power differentials between men and women in the outside world and the ways that these mystify the treatment or consultation context should be part of any assessment of problems.

Gender differences between clients and helpers form a salient feature of the macrosystem. Such differences tend to be either dismissed as unimportant or exaggerated to women's detriment, as when single-parent women are told they must have male helpers for their children. Rather, such differences need to be confirmed and examined for the part they play in the family–larger system relationship.

Interventions are required that serve to empower women, that focus on interdependent relationship options, and that realign women's positions vis-à-vis their families and the larger systems.

Larger systems are the transmitters of our culture's assumptions and fundamental values regarding human beings, their need for care, locus of blame, and responsibility for change. If unexamined or unquestioned, a patriarchal process reflective of the culture at large is easy for larger systems to support. Work with families and larger systems that is sensitive to women's issues will avoid perpetuating patterns that are detrimental to women and will introduce patterns that facilitate empowerment and equality of experience and opportunity.

CHAPTER 8

Consulting to Larger Systems

A recent and developing trend in the work of skilled family therapists has been to respond to requests for consultations from larger systems (Wynne, McDaniel & Weber, 1986). This chapter addresses such consultations as they occur in large human service systems, including mental health clinics, hospitals, public schools, welfare, and specialized programs for particular population groups.

While many of the assessment, interviewing and intervention techniques described above are useful when consulting to larger systems, certain differences between family systems and human service systems must be borne in mind. While family members have a shared intergenerational history and probably a shared future, human service systems' members do not. Staff turnover is frequently high in these systems, and changes in leadership are frequent. Members of such systems are often confronted with loyalty issues regarding changing leadership and must deal with attachments in a temporary sphere.

While family decision-making practices are generally available for examination due to members' proximity, larger systems are embedded in complex bureaucratic structures that are vested with decision-making powers such that a sense of immediacy and opportunity to influence decision making is absent. Workers in human service systems frequently experience a sense of apathy and cynicism while attempting the difficult job of ameliorating apathy and cynicism in clients. A consultant entering a large system may be greeted with similar apathy and cynicism and must take care to place this in its larger sociopolitical context.

While many families may communicate with mixed messages, the mixed message in large human service systems is unique; it centers on the opposing and dualistic mandates of such systems, involving care giving on the one hand and social control on the other. These mandates, which frequently confuse the clients of such systems, also often confuse the workers in their daily interactions with each other and with clients. In addition, what may be seen as care giving by the larger system may, in fact, be experienced as social control by the clients.

THE CONSULTANT'S ENTRY

As one enters a larger system, one is, in fact, entering a new culture with norms, values, beliefs, legal requirements, and world views that may be unfamiliar. The consultant must enter with respect for this new culture if participants are to share their issues and concerns candidly.

Requests for consultation to a larger system may come from various levels within the system. Just as one moves carefully in responding to a request for family therapy, in order to maximize one's influence with the system, so one must move carefully in negotiating a consulting contract. Several questions should shape the consultant's activities initially.

1. Why is a consultation being sought now?
2. Is consultation an invitation for systemic change or an invitation to help maintain the status quo?
3. Who in the system agrees and who disagrees with the need for consultation?
4. Does the system have a history of utilizing consultants? If so, what were the topics or areas of prior consultations, and what were the outcomes?
5. Are people hopeful or cynical about consultation?
6. Who is to be involved? Is the consultant being asked by one part of the system to fix another part of the system, in a way that bears similarities to parents who send a child to therapy but will not entertain systemic change?

Such questions focus the consultant on interactional and organizational issues and avoid the traps of triangulation and blame.

One should enter the larger system seeking resources rather than deficiencies and affirming the participants as the best sources of information about the system. If one is following a long list of prior failed consultations, it is especially advisable to avoid appearing too expert. The complementary one-down position is useful upon entering the larger system. In many larger systems, consultation has become one piece of a larger, repetitive pattern, resulting in no change. One's first area of interest, just as with families who have had lots of helpers, is to discern this pattern, make it overt, and design new and unexpected methods of entry and ongoing work that will not replicate prior failures.

Consultants working with larger systems should carefully avoid relating to the system in ways that replicate the system's major difficulties. It is not unusual, for instance, that a system marked by tentative decision making will engender similar tentativeness in the entering consultant or that a system marked by a high degree of conflict soon finds itself struggling with its consultant. Since systemic change requires difference at a pattern level, it is crucial that the consultant not replicate patterns within the system at the larger system–consultant interface.

ASSESSMENT

Consultation to a larger system involves initial assessment of intrasystem and intersystem issues that involve the larger system and its clients, the larger system and other larger systems, the larger system and the community, or any combination of these.

Intrasystem Issues

Several dimensions inform the assessment of intrasystem issues. The first involves definitions of the problem and includes the following questions: (1) Who in the system is defining a problem requiring consultation? (2) What are the elements of the problem? (3) For whom is it a problem? (4) For whom is it not a problem? (5) Who first identified the problem? (6) Who talks to whom about it? (7) Are there other problems that some people identify as more pressing than the one for which consultation is being sought? (8) How has the system solved similar problems? (9) How would things be different if this problem were solved? While these questions focus the consultant and the participants, they also begin to impart information to the consultant regarding alliances, splits, myths, and staff expectations of the consultant.

The second dimension involves examining the system's cherished beliefs and labels. The way a system views itself may be incongruent with interactional actualities, and this may result in a distorted perception of staff participation. For instance, an agency may insist that it is a nonhierarchical organization when in fact key decisions are being made by a small cadre that excludes the rest of the staff. While cherished beliefs will often become apparent, it may be useful to ask some of the following questions: (1) What is most important about this agency? (2) What do you most want to be known for? (3) How are decisions made or policies changed? (4) How do you understand your mandate? (5) How are you seen by clients? (6) How are you seen by other agencies? (7) How are you seen by the public?

As the agency's beliefs about itself, its functional purpose, its structures, and so on, are verbalized, the consultant is able to observe how well these match the system's actual operations. It may emerge that one or more members hold beliefs that are antithetical to the majority and hence may be getting squeezed to conform. The system may show itself to have little or no tolerance for difference, and it may require subterfuge to belong. Conversely, the agency may have no strong belief system at all, resulting in a lack of connectedness and loyalty among participants.

The third area involves determining the system's preferred locus of blame for its difficulties. Does the agency blame one person and see all solutions dependent on that person's exit? It so, one will often find a pattern of extrusion as the solution to problems. Is blame placed outside on some amorphous system? Do staff members blame themselves and feel demoralized? Are clients of the agency blamed for not performing according to the agency's mandate? Is blame static or shifting? Often, staff members will not discuss blame directly, and the consultant must devise questions to elicit this information. Such questions might include: (1) How do you explain why this is happening? (2) What do you think needs to change for this to be solved? The answers to these questions often reveal where blame is being placed. The tone with which such questions are answered may also indicate morale level and issues of self-blame.

Intersystem Issues

Human service systems operate in relationship to many other systems. These other systems must be considered in the consultant's search for the meaningful system for intervention. Three major areas must be assessed. The first involves the agency's relationships with the clients it serves. Human service systems exist by virtue of providing a service to clients, and hence these relationships are crucial to agency functioning. The consultant's assessment should include the following: (1) Do staff view their relationships with clients as positive or negative, as generally successful or failing, as accomplishing the agency's mandate or not? (2) Do staff feel a sense of satisfaction from their work with clients or not? (3) Do staff feel angry with clients? If so, what percentage of the time? (4) Do staff appear interested in gaining new skills for work with clients? (5) Do staff worry about particular clients for great quantities of time when they are not at work? Questions such as these will reveal patterns of overinvolvement, burnout, low morale, and so on, or such themes as optimism or hope.

The second area involves the complex relationships between this agency and other human service–provider systems. In any given community, the mental health clinic, the probation department, children's protective services, and so on, all interact with one another. Such interaction is generally about particular clients but may also be about funding, the service mandate, or staffing patterns. It is not unusual for the consultant to discover very difficult and troubled relationships marked by mistrust, fear of scarcity of resources, blame for failed cases, frustration over lack of agreement, and so on. The consultant who ignores these complexities may inadvertently contribute to their escalation. Thus, the consultant must attend to the potential impact on multiple systems, even if only one system has a designated consultant.

The consultant's assessment should include the following: (1) What agencies do you regularly interact with? (2) Which agencies do you consider as your allies? (3) Which agencies do you have regular difficulties with? What is the nature of such difficulties? How are such difficulties approached or solved? The answers to these questions, and the tone with which they are answered, will inform the consultant regarding patterned alliance and splits, escalating symmetry regarding shared cases, and the myths and beliefs regarding other agencies. One will also discover whether agencies that regularly struggle with each other occasionally submerge their differences in regard to a particular family or if there are situations in which families remain in the human service network by virtue of being the intense focus of conflict between two or more agencies. The questions help the agency to experience its connectedness to other systems and begin to raise the possibilities of networking strategies.

The third area involves the agency's relationship to the larger community, to the public that funds the agency through taxation. The agency's relationships to the community are often ignored, yet this may be an arena of great stress. Often human service systems are given a profoundly mixed message by the larger community that simultaneously desires that the job be done yet shows a lack of respect for those who do it. Clients (e.g., probationers, the elderly, the handicapped, welfare recipients, etc.) served by human service systems are often not highly regarded by the community. Hence, the public often regards success with these clients as a form of control rather than something that facilitates their development. The consultant must be aware of this often hidden source of stress that involves a sense of being unappreciated and poorly esteemed for one's work.

In addition, specific human service systems may have particular difficulties with the larger community; an example might be a chronic aftercare project that wishes to establish a group home in a residential neighborhood. In such a situation, the unit for consultation may well be the agency *and* neighborhood residents.

The consultant's assessment should include the following: (1) How do you think the community regards your agency? (2) How do you think the community regards your clients? (3) What would constitute success in your work for the community? Does this match or differ with your own view of success? (4) Have there been particular disputes with the community? How have these been approached? What has been the outcome? The responses to these questions will let the consultant begin to understand the nature of the relationship between the agency and the community. One will discern if there is a high degree of mistrust and misunderstanding between the agency and the community. One may discover extremely rigid boundaries, or one may find that community members participate in decision making of the agency as members of a board. The questions also help to raise the agency's own sense of its embeddedness in a wider context that affects its functioning.

In examining the various aspects of intersystem relationships, the consultant seeks to discover how others see the agency, how the agency believes it is regarded by others, and the ways in which such relationships affect the agency's overall functioning. This information helps the consultant determine the correct level for intervention (Imber-Black, 1986b).

TYPES OF CONSULTATIONS

Consultations to large human service systems, categorized on the basis of the initial consultation request, include case-based, relationship-based, education- or in-service-based, and program development–based. Education-based consultations most often include aspects of program development, and the two categories will be considered together. Some consultations may, of course, include more than one of these areas or may over the course of the consultation develop from one area to another. While these consultation types are entry points, the consultant should guard against deciding unilaterally that an agency needs another type of consultation or moving from one type to another without frank and open discussion with all concerned.

In a case-based consultation, a request is made by a larger system for consultation on a particularly problematic case or a group of cases that share common elements. Upon entry into the system, the consultant may discover that the complaint about the case is usefully conceptualized the way a symptom is conceptualized in family treatment. Individuals, agency subsystems, and whole agencies often organize in response to issues in stuck cases. A useful consultation seeks to introduce second-order change that will obviate the need for future consultation requests on identical topics. Case-based consultations may take the form of a family–larger system interview as described in previous chapters; however, it is useful for the consultant to inquire about the usualness of the problem being presented, for instance when an agency describes an issue of anger between clients and larger system or a repeating triangle between the system seeking consultation, another larger system, and various client systems. If a repetitive pattern is confirmed, then the consultation should address issues at this level and not simply seek to resolve the issues regarding one family.

A community mental health system providing outpatient services sought consultation regarding a family whose therapy was protracted and unsuccessful. Initial entry into the mental health system revealed a long-standing conflict with the local child-welfare office that played out in a number of shared cases, of which the case under discussion happened to be one. A pattern emerged that included conflictual triangulation of clients, such that shared cases frequently created clients who were in a loyalty bind: they were being asked to form primary alliances with workers from each system, who were, in fact, in conflict with each other. The exact content of the conflict seemed to center on a symmetrical escalation regarding whose mandate was more important, disagreements over sharing information regarding clients who had given consent for shared information, and status in the community. The child-welfare system referred cases grudgingly to the mental health system. The mental health system viewed itself as the rescuer of families from the child-welfare system and frequently lost maneuverability thereby. Relationships between the two larger systems had deteriorated to the point where they seldom met with each other. Relationships were extremely formalistic, and gossip was rife. Since the community being served was within a small city, the two systems were forced to interact regarding certain clients.

Upon discerning this pattern, the consultant began by coaching the mental health director in order to establish a meeting between the two larger systems. The agenda for the meeting was to discuss the case for which consultation had initially been sought and to begin to discuss similar cases in order to bring the pattern involving such cases into awareness. As case after case was discussed, the participants from mental health and child welfare began to see the triangle. Gradually, the consultant was able to ask other questions regarding the work of each system and the relationship between the two larger systems. Ways in which the developmental mandate of the mental health system often conflicted with the social control mandate of the child-welfare system were discussed for the first time. Myths that each system had about the other were called into question. Future-oriented questions that posed a different relationship between the two systems were raised in order to break the stalemate. Towards the end of the meeting, the original case that had prompted the consultation was raised by the consultant, and the participants were asked to make a plan that would detriangulate the family. The plan included agreements about what information was appropriate to share, based on agency mandates and family consent, and what information belonged within the boundaries of the family's relationship with one or the other larger system. This was the first time that the two larger systems had not allowed their discussions regarding shared clients to deteriorate.

Following this meeting, the consultant held a family–larger system session with the representatives of the two systems and the family in question, in order to clarify roles and boundaries. The family members stated that they had been very confused in their work with the two larger systems, particularly regarding whose role was what, who to turn to in crisis, what the parameters of success were with each system, and so on. They were quite aware of the conflict between the two systems, even though this had never been discussed openly, and the father remarked that it made him wonder how he could get help for his very conflictual family when the helpers were fighting with each other. The session ended with specific agreements on goals for the family's work with each system and a written contract regarding what information should be shared between the larger systems and how feedback to the family was to occur.

The next and final step in this consultation involved the consultant meeting again with representatives of both larger systems. The workers on the shared case were asked to report on their family–larger system interview. An initial working agreement regarding other cases was then developed that spelled out boundaries and appropriate complementarities between the two systems. A quarterly review of the agreement was included.

The consultant's final intervention was to urge that each system offer in-service training to the other, in order to diminish myths between the two systems and to organize a relationship in which each system's work was valued.

The consultant followed up in 1 year and found that the two larger systems were largely cooperative, that they knew when to meet on problematic cases, and that the prior pattern of triangulation with families had disappeared. Each system had offered in-service training to the other regarding their mandates.

Requests for relationship-based consultations are made when workers within a given larger system are experiencing difficulties in their relationships with one another. Examples include complaints of low morale, two or more staff members relating with a high degree of conflict, symptomatic expression by one or more people, patterns of inappropriate secrecy and covert alliances, and staff burnout. Blame-oriented hypotheses are often rife, as participants struggle in their relationships with one another. In extreme situations the daily work of the agency takes a distant second place to the energy being expended on relationship problems.

The consultant's entry in relationship-based consultations requires careful analysis of the larger system in order to obviate being seen as the ally of one of the conflicting parties. Consultation regarding staff relations is often sought after a situation has gone from bad to worse. Prior solutions, the preferred focus of blame, and patterns of scape-goating should be investigated in order to begin to reframe the situation.

BRIEF EXAMPLE: THE SYSTEMIC FUNCTION OF RELATIONSHIP CONFLICTS

Consultation was sought by a multiservice system because two supervisors were not getting along with one another. In this system, one supervisor was in charge of a mental health unit and the other was in charge of a child-welfare unit. Their relationship was rapidly deteriorating, and their respective staffs, as might be expected, were taking sides. Personal blame was rife and resulted in mutual accusations and recriminations. Client care was beginning to suffer. Most of those who assessed the situation from within the organization saw it as a personality problem and believed that one or the other of the supervisors would have to leave. Such individual blame–oriented framing is common when relationship issues are targeted by larger systems. Investigation from a systemic perspective yielded a very different picture. The two units had been separate entities until recently, when by administrative fiat a multiservice organization was created. Most workers were very unsettled by this change. At the upper levels, far removed from this particular agency, battles ensued regarding the meaning of the merger, the future of each group's service mandate, and where power would reside. The two supervisors attended high-level administrative meetings, but each chose to protect the staff members from knowledge of the current chaos. Thus their struggles with one another were a metaphor for interactions in central administration and a distraction for their staffs during a highly unstable time.

The consultant was able to reframe their alleged conflict as a cooperative effort to protect their staffs and an effort to discover solutions that were not being found at higher levels. Following this initial reframing of the issues, the consultant worked with each supervisor to develop a plan for greater openness with the staff regarding the current problems in the larger system. As such openness ensued, rumors abated. The focus of each staff shifted from the relationship between the supervisors to what could be done within the constraints of the new mandate.

Larger public-sector systems have increasingly turned to family therapists for education-based consultation. The consultant is asked in to give in-service training to all or part of a staff. Such consultations are often more complicated than they may first appear and should not be simply regarded as teaching requests. A workshop or series of seminars given in a larger system is an *intervention* in that system. It is important for the consultation to discern where the request is coming from, who thinks it's important to learn the material, and what sort of commitment to working in a new way is being made. It is also important for the consultant not to proselytize. Not every larger system should do family therapy. A consultant can effectively impart understanding of systemic process that will enhance an agency's functioning, rather than turning it into a family therapy program.

BRIEF EXAMPLE: A GROUP HOME LEARNS ABOUT FAMILIES AND SYSTEMS

An agency that provided group homes for mentally handicapped young adults who were leaving home for the first time sought education-based consultation regarding family process. As the consultant began, it became clear that the request for consultation arose out of repeated problems that staff were having interacting with the parents of clients. The request for information about family process indicated the group home staff's conceptualization of the locus of the problem *in* the families. The consultant began by meeting this request. She focused on family life-cycle issues, highlighting the leaving-home phase of development and its special proportions for families with mentally handicapped members whom they may never have anticipated leaving home. During this presentation, the consultant discovered that the group home expected a very rigid boundary to develop between the group home and the clients' families. Such a rigid boundary was in marked contrast to the leaving-home phase of development of nonhandicapped young adults, who generally maintain contact with and influences from their families. In short, clients were expected to completely switch their loyalties from their families to the group home. Families were expected to distance, have formal visits, and not intrude. Those families who insisted on more contact were stipulated as overinvolved. When problems ensued, the parents were asked to seek therapy.

    The consultant began to ask questions regarding the relationship between the group home staff and families *prior* to the client moving to the group home. What emerged was a pattern in which the parents were given information about the group home. The group home did not elicit information from the parents regarding their special knowledge of their children. No effort was made to affirm the parents' many years of expertise as the care provider for their handicapped child. Rather than defining a working partnership between group home and family, the agency had attempted to initiate complementary relationships in which they had all the professional expertise regarding working with mentally handicapped people, and the parents were to be the recipients of such knowledge.

During this discussion, the staff highlighted case after case of problematic relationships with families and the difficult behavior of clients who were, as it turned out, caught in the triangles between family and agency.

Following the educational input, the consultant began to raise what she framed as "programmatic experiments." It was suggested that for the next five new clients, a special effort be made to involve the family in the transition from home to group home. Workers were instructed in methods to interview the parents regarding effective ways to work with the young adults, thus affirming the parents' years of experience, and regarding their experiences with larger systems in their child's behalf, in order to establish a different relationship with the group home staff. Staff met regularly with the consultant during the experiment. They reported being astounded at the information they gathered about the families' relationships to other larger systems, as they heard many painful stories of disqualification and disappointment. All of the families were eager to tell what they had experienced. The staff began to discover a qualitative difference in the entry process and settling in of the clients. Relationships between staff and families were markedly better, as a less rigid boundary was established and the parents were affirmed for their contributions, rather than kept at a distance.

The group home followed the experiment with the establishment of policies that involved families in the transition from home to group home and that encouraged rather than discouraged contact.

In this consultation, an initial request for education arose from an ongoing relationship problem. The consultant met the educational request and utilized this as a springboard for broader systems change that enhanced agency, client, and family relationships. At no time was it suggested that the group home implement family therapy. Rather, by educating the staff about family development *and* family–larger systems relationships, the group home processes changed vis-à-vis families.

Sometimes education-based requests mask relationship issues within a larger system. For instance, a symmetrical struggle between two subsystems with a larger system may be at the heart of an education-based consultation request. The consultant needs to know the history of how this system deals with new ideas. The system's typical response to difference will be operative in education-based consultation.

Education-based consultation to large human service systems must be executed in ways that affirm existing competencies. For instance, to ignore the psychodynamic expertise of a mental health staff while introducing family systems competencies is to invite resistance to the consultation and to contribute to unnecessary staff splits.

Requests to help implement family therapy within existing systems should be approached with caution. It is especially important for the consultant to assess the whole larger system, examine the meaning and timing of the request, and avoid unplanned alliances that disqualify the theoretical positions of other components of the larger system and contribute to symmetrically escalating patterns between subsystems regarding which approach is best.

It is not unusual for education-based consultations to broaden into program-development consultations. As people in the larger system begin to see the implications of the new learning, program-development requirements begin to emerge. At this juncture, it is important for the consultant to be sensitive to the demands and intricacies of the larger system, as program development often requires major systemic changes.

BRIEF EXAMPLE: ESTABLISHING A FAMILY THERAPY PROJECT
WITHIN A PUBLIC SCHOOL SYSTEM

An education-based consultation was requested by the director of special education for a medium-sized school district. The request was for family therapy training for the guidance staff involved with special education students. At the beginning of the consultation, the entire guidance staff was required by the director to attend the sessions. Interest in learning a new way of working with students, their families, and the school system was high. However, as the consultation proceeded many issues of how to implement the new material emerged. At this juncture, what began as an education-based consultation shifted to a program-development consultation. While continuing the educational in-service with the staff, the consultant met frequently with the director of special education to examine the feasibility of the guidance staff offering family therapy services within the school system. Criteria for such services were established in order to obviate competition with the local mental health clinic. Students and families whose difficulties were clearly school related became the population for the project. Operating between the family and the classroom enabled the counselors to reframe students' problems as interactional and systemic, thus reducing individual blame. Armed with systems concepts, the counselors were able to be "shuttle diplomats" in situations where tension was high between the family and the school. Where ongoing family therapy ensued, family privacy was protected by holding meetings in buildings other than the one the student attended.

The consultant continued to meet with the director of special education approximately quarterly over a 4-year period, in order to continue with the program development. These meetings also insured that the consultant understood the special education context within which the project was developing. Monthly case-based consultations were held with the guidance staff. During this time the project developed from in-service training in family therapy to an experimental program offering services to families with school-related problems, and finally to an established family therapy project within the school district, which included a commitment to video and live supervision and the availability of counselor consultations to teachers in order to intervene in classroom problems. It is important to note that the major program-development thrust of this consultation occurred during a time of severe budget cutbacks within the school district. Initially, the staff felt discouraged, but the consultation focused on what was still possible, despite the budget constraints. Staff morale was maintained by a joint commitment to the project and by problem solving that bypassed budget constraints through creative uses of time, a willingness to work in less than optimal conditions (including initially conducting family sessions in the only space available—an old locker room) and demonstrations of efficacy, which ultimately led to greater institutional support.

CONCLUSION

Consultation to larger systems is a complex activity, requiring the capacity to move among levels of a system, to understand that system's embeddedness in several outside contexts, to appreciate and utilize systemic patterns, and to function collaboratively with the larger system. Effective consultation focuses on the development of resources within the larger system and seeks to enhance existing competencies, while imparting new information and facilitating systemic change.

Coda. Families, Larger Systems, and the Wider Social Context: Personal Reflections and Questions

My journey in the family–larger system labyrinth has led increasingly to the social, political, and economic contexts in which families and larger systems are embedded. I believe attention to this broader level is required in order to prevent even excellent family–larger system work from becoming that which simply makes everything go more smoothly within a wider context that ultimately disempowers a significant portion of the population. Increasingly, so-called "multiproblem" families, while most often multi–larger system families (Selig, 1976), are also most often poor families. The culture that requires their poverty cannot be ignored in a family–larger system analysis.

While the primary call of this work has expanded our concepts of assessment and intervention from the family level to the family–larger system level for clinical work with all families, I believe this shift is especially profound for public-sector work, which most often involves poor families and the larger systems with which such families interact. As a therapist and trainer working with a family–larger system point of view, my attention here is drawn to such larger systems as public welfare, child welfare, public hospitals, public schools, and shelters.

The relationship between poor families and workers in those larger systems whose *raison d'être* is to help the poor, rather than to alleviate poverty, is especially poignant. Families and helpers alike are frequently disempowered, unable to effect lasting change in the macrosystem.

A little boy who has lived in 10 foster homes in 5 years says, "I've had so many . . . workers I can't remember them all. They say, 'All right, we're gonna help you, we're gonna help you.' A million times the . . . workers say, 'We're on your side.' But then they go against you. They're always on your back. It's almost like Rambo against the Vietcong"

(Rimer, 1987). A worker in this same system, where turnover in one year is 80%, talks of having to "put her life on hold" in order to do the job. Here a child, whose future will no doubt involve relationships with multiple helpers, envisions those relationships in militaristic metaphors in a country whose conservative agenda clearly values spending for war preparation over spending for a child's life, and a worker is on the road to burning out.

The proximity of poor families and helpers in the macrosystem, coupled with their mutual distance from those decision makers with the power to effect real change in the distribution of resources, contributes to a relationship often marked by misdirected anger and tension, by reciprocal mistrust, and by cynicism.

Thus, as I begin to examine the family–larger system relationship, including my own place in it, I am led directly to the wider social context that organizes and shapes a given family's view of itself, the larger system's mandates, and the possibilities of work I and others may be able to facilitate. It is this wider context that currently lacks any coherent family policy and so enables the creation of larger systems that often fragment families while simultaneously espousing a right-wing rhetoric glorifying a mythical family that never needs outside help. It is this wider context that continues to allow many public schools to inadequately educate poor and minority children and to inappropriately channel many of these children into special education classes. It is this wider context that disallows access to adequate health care for a significant portion of the population. It is this wider context that has led in recent years to what one client referred to as a "growth industry," those larger systems whose mandate is to work with the problems caused by homelessness, while policy makers and politicians continue to eschew the primary solution needed, which is adequate low-cost housing for all. The exquisite, yet most often invisible, connection between family members, helpers, complex personal and interpersonal problems, and the social, economic, and political context compel our attention, for intervention at the wrong level of the macrosystem runs the risk of perpetuating rather than alleviating human suffering.

In this present work, I have focused on methods for the therapist to develop new and unanticipated relationships with families who have had chronically unsuccessful relationships with larger systems, and on methods to repair family–larger system relationships in ways that may lead to empowerment of family members and helpers alike. The work has made me aware of a certain ironic possibility that my focus on altering iatrogenic effects will require yet another specialist in an already crowded macrosystem! My ongoing fear as I have developed the present work has been that a well-crafted set of family–larger system assessment and intervention skills may, at times, unwittingly assist in maintaining the status quo at the next level of the macrosystem. Thus, attention to the effects of our work at the next level of the macrosystem is required. At the same time, attention to the effects of family–larger system work on ourselves as therapists and consultants is also needed.

The more family–larger system work that I do, the more I am drawn to collaborative and nonhierarchical models of practice, both between other workers and myself and between family members and myself. This work nurtures my hopefulness that the expansion in our vision of practice possibilities from the individual, to the family, to the family and larger system, with its concomitant shifts from sole practitioner to collaborative teams, will lead next to our discovery of effective ways to address problems and issues at the level of the wider social context.

This direction makes me feel both humble and exhilarated. My sense of the interdependence of families, workers in larger systems, and myself, when I have been allowed to enter this relationship, has been deepened by this work, as I am increasingly aware that none of us are empowered unless all of us are.

References

Aponte, H. (1976). The family–school interview: An eco-structural approach. *Family Process, 15,* 303–312.

Auerswald, E. H. (1968). Interdisciplinary versus ecological approach. *Family Process, 7,* 202–215.

Bateson, G. (1972). *Steps to an ecology of mind.* New York: Ballantine Books.

Bateson, G. (1979). *Mind and nature: A necessary unity.* New York: E. P. Dutton.

Bell, L. (1982). *Change and resistance in schools: A case study follow-up and general systems analysis of the impact of the federal Title IX project in one school district.* Unpublished doctoral dissertation, University of Massachusetts, Amherst.

Bell, N., & Zucker, R. (1968–1969). Family–hospital relationships in a state hospital setting: A structural–functional analysis of the hospitalization process. *International Journal of Social Psychiatry, 15,* 73–80.

Berger, M. (1984). Social network interventions for families that have a handicapped child. In E. Imber Coppersmith (Ed.), *Families with handicapped members.* Rockville, MD: Aspen Systems.

Bloomfield, S., Neilson, S., & Kaplan, L. (1984). Retarded adults, their families and larger systems: A new role for the family therapist. In E. Imber Coppersmith (Ed.), *Families with handicapped members.* Rockville, MD: Aspen Systems.

Bokos, P. J., & Schwartzman, J. (1985). Family therapy and methadone treatment of opiate addiction. In J. Schwartzman (Ed.), *Families and other systems: The macrosystemic context of family therapy.* New York: Guilford Press.

Carter, E., & McGoldrick Orfanidis, M. (1976). Family therapy with one person and the family therapist's own family. In P. J. Guerin (Ed.), *Family therapy: Theory and practice.* New York: Gardner Press.

Coleman, S. (1983). A Case of non-treatment of a non-problem problem. *Journal of Strategic and Systemic Therapies, 2,* 62–66.

Combrinck-Graham, L., & Higley, L. W. (1984). Working with families of school-aged handicapped children. In E. Imber Coppersmith (Ed.), *Families with handicapped members.* Rockville, MD: Aspen Systems.

Fisch, R., Weakland, J. H., & Segal, L. (1982). *The tactics of change: Doing therapy briefly*. San Francisco: Jossey-Bass.

Goolishian, H., & Anderson, H. (1981). Including non-blood related persons in family therapy. In A. Gurman (Ed.), *Questions and answers in the practice of family therapy*. New York: Brunner/Mazel.

Haley, J. (1976). *Problem solving therapy*. San Francisco: Jossey-Bass.

Harbin, H. T. (1985). The family and the psychiatric hospital. In J. Schwartzman (Ed.), *Families and other systems: The macrosystem context of family therapy*. New York: Guilford Press.

Harkaway, J. (1983). Obesity: Reducing the larger systems. *Journal of Strategic and Systemic Therapies*, *2*, 2–14.

Harrell, F. (1980). Family dependency as a transgenerational process: An ecological analysis of families in crises. Unpublished doctoral dissertation, University of Massachusetts, Amherst.

Hoffman, L., and Long, L. (1969). A systems dilemma. *Family Process*, *8*, 211–234.

Imber-Black, E. (1986a). Odysseys of a learner. In D. Efron (Ed.), *Journeys: Expansion of the strategic–systemic therapies*. New York: Brunner/Mazel.

Imber-Black, E. (1986b). The systemic consultant and human service provider systems. In L. C. Wynne, S. H. McDaniel, and T. T. Weber (Eds.), *Systems consultation: A new perspective for family therapy*. New York: Guilford Press.

Imber-Black, E. (1986c). Toward a resource model in systemic family therapy. In M. Karpel (Ed.), *Family resources: The hidden partner in family therapy*. New York: Guilford Press.

Imber-Black, E. (1986d). Women, families and larger systems. In M. Ault-Riche (Ed.), *Women and family therapy*. Rockville, MD: Aspen Systems.

Imber-Black, E. (1988). Idiosyncratic life cycle transitions and therapeutic rituals. In E. Carter and M. McGoldrick (Eds.), *The family life cycle: A framework for family therapy* (2nd ed.). New York: Gardner Press.

Imber-Black, E. (in press). The mentally handicapped in context. *Family Systems Medicine*.

Imber Coppersmith, E. (1982a). Family therapy in a public school system. In A. Gurman (Ed.), *Questions and answers in the practice of family therapy* (vol. 2). New York: Brunner/Mazel.

Imber Coppersmith, E. (1982b). From hyperactive to normal but naughty: A multi-system partnership in delabeling. *International Journal of Family Psychiatry*, *3*, 131–144.

Imber Coppersmith, E. (1983a). The family and public service systems: An assessment method. In B. Keeney (Ed.), *Diagnosis and assessment in family therapy*. Rockville, MD: Aspen Systems.

Imber Coppersmith, E. (1983b). The family and public sector systems: Interviewing and interventions. *Journal of Strategic and Systemic Therapies*, *2*, 38–47.

Imber Coppersmith, E. (1985a). Families and multiple helpers: A systemic perspective. In D. Campbell and R. Draper (Eds.), *Applications of systemic family therapy*. New York: Grune & Stratton.

Imber Coppersmith, E. (1985b). Teaching trainees to think in triads. *Journal of Marital and Family Therapy*, *11*, 61–66.

Imber Coppersmith, E. (1985c). We've got a secret: A non-marital marital therapy. In A. Gurman (Ed.), *Casebook of marital therapy*. New York: Guilford Press.

Karpel, M. A. (1980). Family secrets: I. Conceptual and ethical issues in the relationship context; II. Ethical and practical considerations in therapeutic management. *Family Process, 19*, 295–306.

Lederer, W. J., & Jackson, D. D. (1968). *The mirages of marriage*. New York: Norton.

Lee, J. (1980). The helping professional's use of language in describing the poor. *American Journal of Orthopsychiatry, 50*, 580–584.

MacKinnon, L., & Marlett, N. (1984). A social action perspective: The disabled and their families in context. In E. Imber Coppersmith (Ed.), *Families with handicapped members*. Rockwell, MD: Aspen Systems.

Madanes, C. (1981). *Strategic family therapy*. San Francisco: Jossey-Bass.

Miller, D. (1983). Outlaws and invaders: The adaptive function of alcohol abuse in the family-helper supra system. *Journal of Strategic and Systemic Therapies, 2*, 15–27.

Minuchin, S. (1974). *Families and family therapy*. Cambridge: Harvard University Press.

Minuchin, S., & Fishman, H. C. (1981). *Family therapy techniques*. Cambridge: Harvard University Press.

Morawetz, A., & Walker, G. (1984). *Brief therapy with single parent families*. New York: Brunner/Mazel.

Moynihan, D. P. (1965). *The Negro family: A case for national action*. Washington DC: U.S. Government Printing Office.

New York Times, (1987, March 19). B. 9.

Papp, P. The Greek chorus and other techniques of paradoxical therapy. *Family Process, 19*, 45–57.

Paul, N. L., & Bloom, J. D. (1970). Multiple-family therapy: Secrets and scapegoating in family crisis. *International Journal of Group Psychychotherapy, 20*, 37–47.

Pincus, L., & Dare, C. (1978). *Secrets in the family*. New York: Pantheon Books.

Pogrebin, L. C. (1983). *Family politics: Love and power on an intimate frontier*. New York: McGraw Publishers.

Rimer, S. (1987, March 19). A foster child's nightmare: Moving 10 times in 5 years. *New York Times*, pp. A-1, B-9.

Roberts, J. (1984). Families with infants and young children who have special needs. In E. Imber Coppersmith (Ed.)., *Families with handicapped members*. Rockville, MD: Aspen Systems.

Sarason, S. B., and Doris, J. (1979). *Educational handicap, public policy, and social history: A broadened perspective on mental retardation*. New York: Free Press.

Schwartzman, H., and Kneifel, A. W. (1985). Familiar institutions: How the child care system replicates family patterns. In J. Schwartzman (Ed.), *Families and other systems: The macrosystemic context of family therapy*. New York: Guilford Press.

Schwartzman, J., and Restivo, R. J. (1985). Acting out and staying in: Juvenile probation and the family. In J. Schwartzman (Ed.), *Families and other systems: The macrosystemic context of family therapy.* New York: Guilford Press.

Selig, A. (1976). The myth of the multi-problem family. *American Journal of Orthopsychiatry, 46*, 526–531.

Selvini Palazzoli, M., Boscolo, L., Cecchin, G., and Prata, G. (1978a). *Paradox and counterparadox.* New York: Aronson.

Selvini Palazzoli, M., Boscolo, L., Cecchin, G., and Prata, G. (1978b). A ritualized prescription in family therapy: Odd days and even days. *Journal of Marriage and Family Counseling, 4*, 3–9.

Selvini Palazzoli, M., Boscolo, L., Cecchin, G., and Prata, G. (1980a). Hypothesizing, circularity, neutrality: Three guidelines for the conductor of the session. *Family Process, 19*, 3–12.

Selvini Palazzoli, M., Boscolo, L., Cecchin, G., and Prata, G. (1980b). The problem of the referring person. *Journal of Marital and Family Therapy, 6*, 3–9.

Tomm, K. (1984a). One perspective on the Milan systemic approach: Part I. Overview of development, theory, and practice. *Journal of Marital and Family Therapy, 10*, 113–125.

Tomm, K. (1984b). One perspective on the Milan systemic approach: Part II. Description of session format, interviewing style, and interventions. *Journal of Marital and Family Therapy, 10*, 253–271.

Tomm, K., Lannaman, J., and McNamee, S. (1983, Fall). No interview today: A consultation team intervenes by not intervening. *Journal of Strategic and Systemic Therapies, 2*, 48–61.

Watzlawick, P., Beavin, J. H., and Jackson, D. D. (1967). *Pragmatics of human communications: A study of interactional patterns, pathologies and paradoxes.* New York: Norton.

Watzlawick, P., Weakland, J., and Fisch, R. (1974). *Change: Principles of problem formation and problem resolution.* New York: Norton.

Webb-Woodard, L., and Woodard, B. (1983, Fall). The larger system in the treatment of incest. *Journal of Strategic and Systemic Therapies, 2*, 28–37.

Webb-Woodard, L. (1980). *Selfhood: Discovery of survival values in low income black families in Hartford, Connecticut. Two cases using family systems theory.* Unpublished doctoral dissertation, University of Massachusetts, Amherst.

Wynne, L. C., McDaniel, S. H., and Weber, T. T. (1986). *Systems consultation: A new perspective for family therapy.* New York: Guilford Press.

Index